Health Begins in Him

Biblical Steps to Optimal Health and Nutrition

by
Terry Dorian, Ph.D.

Huntington House Publishers

Huntington House Publishers
P.O. Box 53788
Lafayette, Louisiana 70505

Library of Congress Card Catalog Number 94-79916
ISBN 1-56384-081-2

All Scripture is New American Standard
unless otherwise noted.

Dedication

To Gary, my husband and dearest friend, whose discipline, order, strength, and dignity have shaped my life, whose love and faithfulness is God's daily provision, whose trust and trustworthiness is a treasure, whose dedication as a father is an ever-unfolding blessing of God.

To our children, Jessica Allison, Canaan Dira, Christian Dikran and Jenna Campbell whose faith and faithfulness, love and tenderness, joy, and gladness define my life, whose very lives testify of God's miracles and mercy.

To our daughters and sons-in-law Kimberly Alice and Darren Lancaster and Stacey Anne and Patrick Dee; to Kim and Stacey whose lives impacted mine in ways only God can know, whose open hearts challenged my faith, and whose hopes became my prayers. And to their husbands, Darren Lancaster and Patrick Dee, our delight as sons-in-law, men of virtue, honor, and moral purity chosen by God from the foundation of the earth to bless our lives.

To our children's children, may they glorify God and enjoy Him forever.

To my mother, Elouise C. Hicks whose unconditional love, generosity, and dedication are always with me.

To my father, the late Wiley H. Hicks, who struggled and sacrificed to protect and to provide for our family, who became my precious friend in Christ, who is safe forever in the arms of God.

To our Lord and Savior, Jesus Christ. Blessed be the Father, the Son, and the Holy Ghost, whose song I sing, whose love I know, whose mercy endureth forever. Blessed be the Name of the Lord.

What others have said about *Health Begins in Him*:

As a Board Certified Family Physician and homeschooling father of eight children, I have long had a concern for the nutritional aspects of health.

I have found *Health Begins in Him* to be an excellent source of nutritional information that is presented in an easily understood form and is exceptionally well researched. The practical suggestions and step-by-step approaches for eating nutritiously are the best and most comprehensive I have seen.

Many of the treatment regimens suggested, while certainly outside the venue of mainstream medicine, deserve consideration.

This book should be in the library of any family who has a concern for their nutritional health.

> —Leslie Emhof, M.D., Board Certified Family Physician and home-schooling father of eight children

Having worked with terminally ill patients for 15 years, I have experienced many miracles through alternative therapies, especially nutrition, but most important to me is the healing of my patients' souls.

Health Begins in Him provides profound information for patients to restore not only their physical well-being, but also to find salvation in Jesus Christ. I will recommend this book to all my patients.

> —Dr. Francisco Contreras R., Surgical Oncologist

Contents

Acknowledgments   7

Part One: Faith for the Journey   9

Part Two: Biblical Steps to Optimal Health
          and Nutrition   63

    Step One
    Become a Thankful and Joyful Person   65

    Step Two
    Enjoy Preparing, Serving, and Eating Foods
    Which Are Essential for Optimal Health   85

    Step Three
    Make Time for Life-Saving,
    Life-Enhancing Activities   141

    Step Four
    Prevent or Cure Degenerative Disease   155

Step Five
Present Your Bodies a Living and Holy
Sacrifice: a Prayer and a Benediction   **191**

Notes   **197**

Acknowledgments

With Gratitude

To Dr. Mary Ruth Swope, Dr. Francisco Contreras, Dr. and Mrs. Alfred B. Smith, the Reverend and Mrs. Robert King for their advice, encouragement, and inspiration.

To James Harrison, CEO; Ken Plant, president; Blake, J.B., Peggy, and the other wonderful friends at Magic Mill/Nutriflex for their part in making the study of health and nutrition our family business.

To Frances and Doug Foley who spent weeks in our home helping us attend to our children while I worked on this manuscript, and to Nannie Foley for her prayers.

To Joanne and Fritz Quebe for their faithfulness as friends and for their ministry to our children.

To Melissa and Philip Johnson, and Rene and Kenneth Bumpas for their kindness to our children during this project.

To Sandra and Donald Hicks, Vicki and Robbie Schellhase, Debra and Jim Palmieri, Joyce and James Edwards, Donna and Greg Span, Sue and Brad Becker for their encouragement to wives and workers at home; for sharing their knowledge about milling and baking.

To Jessica, Canaan, Christian, and Jenna who prepared meals, set the house in order, remained cheerful, attended to their studies and blessed our hearts every day of this project.

To Gary whose computer skills and time, talent, diligence, and stamina made this project possible.

Part One

Faith for the Journey

Whoever will call upon the name of the Lord will be saved. How then shall they call upon Him in whom they have not believed? And how shall they believe in Him whom they have not heard? And how shall they hear without a preacher? And how shall they preach unless they are sent? Just as it is written, "How beautiful are the feet of those who bring glad tidings of good things!" However, they did not all heed the glad tidings: for Isaiah says, "Lord, who has believed our report?" So faith comes by hearing and hearing by the word of Christ.

—Romans 10:13–17

O Lord, Thou hast searched me and known me, Thou dost know when I sit down and when I rise up; Thou dost understand my thought from afar. Thou dost scrutinize my path and my lying down. And art intimately acquainted with all my ways. Even before there is a word on my tongue, Behold O Lord, Thou dost know it all. Thou hast enclosed me behind and before, And laid Thy hand upon me. Such knowledge is too wonderful for me; It is too high, I cannot attain it.

Where can I go from Thy Spirit? Or where can I flee from Thy presence? If I ascend to heaven, Thou art there; If I make my bed in Sheol, behold, Thou art there. If I take the wings of the dawn, If I dwell in the remotest part of the sea, Even there Thy hand will lead me. And Thy right hand will lay hold of me. If I say, "Surely the darkness will overwhelm me, And the light around me will be night," Even the darkness is not dark to Thee, And the night is

as bright as the day. Darkness and light are alike to
Thee.

For Thou didst form my inward parts; Thou didst
weave me in my mother's womb. I will give thanks
to Thee, for I am fearfully and wonderfully made;
Wonderful are Thy works, And my soul knows it
very well. My frame was not hidden from Thee,
When I was made in secret, And skillfully wrought
in the depths of the earth. Thine eyes have seen my
unformed substance; And in Thy book they were all
written, The days that were ordained for me, When
as yet there was not one of them.

How precious also are Thy thoughts to me, O God!
How vast is the sum of them! If I should count
them, they would outnumber the sand. When I
awake, I am still with Thee. . . .

Search me, O God, and know my heart; Try me and
know my anxious thoughts; And see if there be any
hurtful way in me, And lead me in the everlasting
way.

                                        —Psalm 139

In 1969, at the age of twenty-two, I walked into a health
food store for the first time. I had no particular concern
about my health, and I did not know that stores, such as
the one that I found off Sunset Drive in South Miami, even
existed. Like many young people, I took my own wellness
for granted. But, that day, as I examined products and
information that were new to me, I realized that numbers
of people had decided to take personal responsibility for
their own health and well-being; they did so primarily by
choosing what to eat and what not to eat.

My own parents enjoyed excellent health. They had
always insisted that we eat regular meals and a "balanced
diet"; but after a few minutes in the health food store, I
realized that I probably knew nothing at all about what
actually constitutes a "balanced diet." As I walked down
the aisles of the store, I saw hundreds of bottles of food
supplements, as well as unfamiliar appliances and food

products. I headed for the book shelves and gathered arm-
loads of books and pamphlets. I was especially interested
in the juice extractors used to produce fresh vegetable
juice from carrots, celery, cabbage, and other vegetables.
At that time I had only been married a few months, and
I wondered if my husband, Frank Bunetta, knew about all
these things. Later that evening, I discovered that he did.
He had patronized health food stores while living in California, and, while working in England, he had vacationed
at several health spas in Europe. He had many experiences
to share. Frank, as my closest friend and mentor, expressed
his delight with my sudden interest in health and healing
through nutrition.

At that time I drank coffee from morning until night.
I smoked over three packages of cigarettes per day. And,
even though it is chilling to remember being young and
lost, I know that it is important to remember. Because in
the remembering I find faith for the journey. Day by day
I know this: Thou dost enlarge my steps under me, And
my feet have not slipped (Ps. 18:3).

I know that He is willing to do the same for every
stranger I meet and for every reader my words reach. The
miracle of John 3:16-21 is for everyone.

In all of our enthusiasm and excitement about life as
we had decided to live it, Frank and I were "dead in our
trespasses and sins." We never imagined whether we were
kind or cold-hearted, brilliant or unimpressive, decent or
decadent. We never thought that we were "by nature children of wrath." We did not know "how" we walked; we
imagined that we energized ourselves.

> And you were dead in your trespasses and sins, in
> which you formerly walked according to the course
> of this world, according to the prince of the power
> of the air, of the spirit that is now working in the
> sons of disobedience.
>
> Among them we too all formerly lived in the lusts
> of our flesh, indulging the desires of the flesh and
> of the mind, and were by nature children of wrath,
> even as the rest. (Eph. 2:1-3)

But, by His grace, I came to recognize smoking cigarettes as both a health hazard and a serious addiction.
Researchers now tell us that nicotine is one of the most
difficult addictions to overcome; and yet, providentially, I
read information which convinced me that I could be free
from the desire to smoke. I also realized that food is a
source of energy and that by eating only "good foods" I
could eliminate my dependency on stimulants. I heard, for
the first time, about cleansing and detoxifying the body.
How very appealing it was to consider feeling lively and to
imagine a kind of physical rebirth. Only by the power of
the Holy Spirit would I come to see my need to be born
again in Him. At that time, I did not acknowledge the need
to worship any "higher being." Neither Frank, nor I, imagined as we journeyed through the darkness that we wor-
shiped spouse, material possessions, and even self. We
thought that we controlled our own lives; we did not know
that we walked "according to the prince of the power of
the air" (Eph. 2:2). And yet, the Lord preserved our lives,
even though we did not seek Him.

Early in high school, I encountered ideas which contradicted the biblical training I had received. From the time
I was six years old, I had attended the North Parkersburg
Baptist Church in Parkersburg, West Virginia. The summer after ninth grade, on the campus of West Virginia
University, during a Speech Institute for High School Students, I heard about the theory of evolution and the philosophy of Ayn Rand. I embraced both. I knew nothing
about the history and the impact of the creation/evolution
conflict. Throughout high school and college, I never heard
an enlightened response to the anti-Christian scientific
theories. I remember vividly what I then perceived to be
the great challenge of life: to create meaning and purpose
in a world which had arrived by chance. During all of my
time in high school and undergraduate school, theater and
the arts defined life for me and offered a means of shaping
reality. But, all of the choices we make lead to chaos when
we do not understand the origin of life and the chief end
of man.

> In the beginning God created the heavens and the earth. In the beginning was the Word, and the Word was with God, and the Word was God. All things came into being by Him, and apart from Him nothing came into being that has come into being. In Him was life, and the life was the light of men. And the light shines in the darkness, and the darkness does not perceive it. (Gen. 1:1; John 1:1–5)

> Whether, then, you eat or drink or whatever you do, do all to the glory of God. (1 Cor. 10:31)

> Whom have I in heaven but Thee? And besides Thee I desire nothing on earth. (Ps. 73:25)

Surely, the first catechism lays a foundation: What is the chief end of man? Man's chief end is to glorify God, and to enjoy Him forever.[1]

But, I had no firm foundation, no revelation of God's Word. When I encountered the current teachings of science and history and listened to the wisdom of the day, I believed only that I had been very ignorant to accept the Christian faith.

> A natural man does not accept the things of the Spirit of God; for they are foolishness to him, and he cannot understand them. (1 Cor. 2:14)

It amazes me now that I developed an interest in health and healing without giving a thought to the One through whom we are "fearfully and wonderfully made" (Ps. 139:14). I did not perceive Him. But, after reading a number of books, I had a consuming interest in learning how to remain fit, and I desperately wanted Frank to remain fit as well. I wanted to know how we could live longer and better.

As Christians, we have a far more powerful motivation than self-preservation. Our bodies are temples of the Holy Spirit.

> Or do you not know that your body is the temple of the Holy Spirit who is in you, whom you have from God, and that you are not your own? For you

have been bought with a price therefore glorify God
in your body. (1 Cor. 6:19)

When you sit down to dine with a ruler, Consider
carefully what is before you; And put a knife to
your throat, If you are a man of great appetite. Do
not desire his delicacies, For it is deceptive food.
(Prov. 23:1–3)

As an unbeliever, seeking information about how to
eat wisely, I did not encounter Christians who advocated
a way of eating which would improve health and reverse
degenerative disease. Certainly such Christians existed; but,
as I later learned, most Christians did not view eating as a
spiritual matter. The Word of God and the power of His
Spirit give every Christian the ability to know what to eat
for health and healing; current scientific research confirms
His Word. And yet, in the name of Christian liberty, God's
people are killing themselves by eating according to the
ways of the world; delicacies are available, affordable, and
desirable. But, the price is high in the end when we eat
"deceptive food" (Prov. 23:3). Our choices have consequences. If we are to do all to the glory of God and to seek
His face regarding every issue of life, surely we must ask
Him what to eat and what not to eat.

I offer a brief record of my own follies and misadven-
tures for the sake of the many people who are facing
various health crises. I have spent hundreds of hours on
the telephone, in workshops, and in private sessions with
women, children, and families in need. Time is precious
for them; they want to avoid detours. They have asked for
a simple book, a sort of primer which will tell them how
to lay a foundation for optimal health. I also trust God's
leading as I give this accounting for an even greater purpose: to proclaim the futility of knowing anything except
Jesus Christ and Him crucified (1 Cor. 2:2). Optimal health
and healing can never occur apart from Christ; walking in
His joy adds a dimension that transcends physical realities.
But, the chief end of man is not to walk in perfect health
or to experience divine healing, it is to know God and to

enjoy Him forever. And, even though people who do not know Him may live long lives and experience good health by adhering to God's natural laws, "what does it profit a man to gain the whole world and forfeit his soul?"

> If anyone wishes to come after Me, let him deny himself, and take up his cross, and follow Me.
>
> For whoever wishes to save his life shall lose it; but whoever loses his life for My sake and the gospel's shall save it.
>
> For what does it profit a man to gain the whole world, and forfeit his soul?
>
> For what shall a man give in exchange for his soul? For whoever is ashamed of Me and My words in this adulterous and sinful generation, the Son of Man will also be ashamed of him when He comes in the glory of His Father with the holy angels. (Mark 8:34–38)

When I married in 1969, I had a foolish confidence that I could preserve the good in our lives and prevent the bad. Moreover, I couldn't discern good and evil, light and dark. I reasoned that eating a proper diet and living in a healthy environment were two ways in which we could live better and longer. I had every encouragement from my husband, Frank, as I sought alternatives to the orthodox views which prevailed in medicine, nutrition, and other fields of study. He himself was a pioneer in the early days of television. At the time we met in 1968 and during the first two years of our marriage, Frank directed the "Jackie Gleason Show" which was produced live before a television audience at the Miami Beach Convention Center. He was fifty-two years old at that time. We were thirty years apart in age. In the very first days of television, Frank worked for Dr. Alan B. DuMont and became the first producer, director, and conceiver of shows for the entire DuMont Network. He explained television to factory workers and to intellectuals who looked back at him with blank faces. Very few people could imagine looking into a "television set" and seeing live action—a virtual window on the world. Frank left school in the ninth grade, worked as the "boy without a body" in a circus act and then as a tool and die maker. He had many different jobs and spent long hours reading in the public library. With Frank, I found an answer to the rebellion of the sixties—an adult who questioned many of the values of his own generation, their standards of behavior, dress, and success. Again, God was there. He knew us in our mothers' wombs and knew that we would be His.

Frank had four brothers who were alive at the time that we married. His oldest brother had died in the summer of 1968, and his mother had died before we met. His father lived with Frank's brother who owned a large waste removal company in Miami. Frank had five sisters, all of whom lived in the Miami area. Frank's daughter and his oldest son are slightly older than I am, and his youngest son is three years younger. Frank had been married twice before our marriage; his children came from his first marriage which began when he was nineteen. Frank and I were kindred spirits, consumed by one another. Now, twenty-five years later, having spent much of my adult life reading history and biography, I understand the danger in that. I would never advise any young person to take the steps I took, but I must carefully acknowledge that God in His infinite mercy rescued me and rescued Frank. To those behind prison bars I have been able to say, with confidence: "The things impossible with men are possible with God" (Luke 18:27). Every man, woman, and child of any age, in any circumstance, can come to know God and enjoy Him forever. Anyone can begin again in Christ!

During the 1969 fall season on the set of the "Gleason Show," a certain photographer spent a lot of time taking shots of Frank with various performers during rehearsals. He often visited our home, accompanied us on various outings, and photographed both Frank and me many times. One day I was looking at some of the shots and I said, "Can't you do something about the darkness under my eyes?" He understood the question. I saw the flaws as the photographer's problem. I will never forget his answer: "Do you know what you're going to look like in a few years if you don't quit smoking?" No, I did not. I hadn't thought about that. I did not consciously think of degeneration, disease, or death as a part of my life. However, his question made me realize that a change in my appearance was imminent. Vanity was probably the strongest motivation for me to quit smoking and to find a way to undo the damage that the smoking had done.

Many of the authors that I began reading during those initial visits to the health food store are still popular today: among them, Dr. N.W. Walker and Bernard Jensen. I was particularly attracted to the ideas and beliefs of the natural hygienists and frugivores. Where did these ideas originate? I searched. The natural hygiene movement began in 1850 with four medical doctors. In 1985, *Fit for Life* by Harvey and Marilyn Diamond popularized the somewhat obscure teachings of this movement. They describe the teachings of natural hygiene as follows:

> The underlying basis of Natural Hygiene is that the body is self-cleansing, self-healing, and self-maintaining. Natural Hygiene is based on the idea that all the healing power of the universe is within the human body; that nature is always correct and cannot be improved upon. Therefore, nature does not seek to thwart any of its own operations. We experience problems of ill health (i.e., excess weight, pain, stress) only when we break the natural laws of life.[2]

The Diamonds' philosophy of healing echoes the authors which I read in 1969 and 1970. Self-determination appealed to me as an unbeliever. Now, through His Word, I know that ill health does not happen "only when we break the natural laws of life" as many writers in this movement may suggest. We were fearfully and wonderfully made by God, and He declares Himself to be our healer. He actually "put" diseases on the Egyptians:

And He said, "If you will give earnest heed to the
voice of the Lord your God, and do what is right in
His sight, and give ear to His commandments, and
keep all His statutes, I will put none of the diseases
on you which I have put on the Egyptians; for I, the
Lord, am your healer." (Exod. 15:26)

The claims supporting a largely raw fruit regime appealed to me in 1969, probably because of the simplicity
of the diet; the harsher, the easier. The notion that human
beings were strict frugivores for millions of years also
seemed reasonable to me before I became a Christian. The
Diamonds' work echoed such teachings in a passage de-
scribing the ideal way to meet the body's needs.

> The ideal percentage of each of the five essentials
> in food as required by the human body is as follows:
> glucose–90%; amino acids–4 to 5%; minerals–3 to
> 4%; fatty acids–1+%; vitamins–under 1%.

> The above represents what the ideal composition of
> food, in terms of the body's needs, would be.

> There is only one food on the planet that fills that
> bill perfectly. It's fruit. This would support Dr. Alan
> Walker's findings that human beings were strict
> frugivores for millions of years. Before we, as a
> race, were led astray by external influences, like all
> other animals in nature we instinctively are what
> most efficiently supplied us with the prerequisites
> of life. In our case this is fruit.[3]

The Word of God does not state that He made man to
be a frugivore or that man departed from such an ideal
diet because he was led astray by "external influences."
Genesis 1:29 records His specific provision: "Then God
said, 'Behold I have given you every plant yielding seed
that is on the surface of all the earth, and every tree which
has fruit yielding seed; it shall be food for you.' " Psalm
104:14 restates that provision. God's provision includes
fruits, vegetables, cereal grasses, and legumes.

Many of the members of the natural hygiene movement contend that not only are meat and dairy harmful,

but grains and beans should be eliminated from the diet as well. The writers whose advice I heeded in 1969 advocated a diet of raw fruits, vegetables, nuts, and seeds. However limited that regime, it offered far more vital nutrients than a diet of devitalized and processed convenience foods, white flour, sugar, and coffee.

As I began studying health and nutrition, it seemed incredible to me that I had never once heard anyone discussing the connection between diet and disease during my entire time in college. At the age of twenty-two, as I considered all of my acquaintances at the undergraduate schools which I attended, I realized that I had never met anyone who had any interest in food beyond being certain that it tasted good. On the other hand, I could think of hundreds of students and faculty members with whom I drank coffee, smoked cigarettes, and ate donuts; I knew that I had spent countless hours enjoying a caffeine-nicotine-white sugar, socially acceptable "high."

My husband, Frank, had stopped smoking years earlier but never suggested that I should quit. He accepted me absolutely unconditionally. However, when I decided to change my lifestyle, he gave me his unqualified support and undivided attention. Even while Frank and I were not yet Christians, his kindness and unselfishness made a wonderful impact on my life. Twenty-five years later, I know that as I minister the love of Christ to my husband and children, friends, acquaintances, and strangers, at some time they will need my unqualified support and undivided attention as well. Time is therefore most precious. Only the Lord can show us how and with whom to spend it.

> So teach us to number our days, That we may present
> to Thee a heart of wisdom. (Ps. 90:12)

Health is about loving and being loved. In my early twenties, I professed love for my parents, younger siblings, my friends, and my spouse—and they professed love for me. But, I knew nothing of His love—agape love—which first fills our hearts and then fills us with love for others—all others.

> The one who does not love does not know God, for
> God is love. By this the love of God was manifested
> in us, that God has sent His only begotten Son into
> the world so that we might live through Him. In this
> is love, not that we loved God, but that He loved us
> and sent His Son to be the propitiation for our sins.
> Beloved, if God so loved us, we also ought to love
> one another. No one has beheld God at any time;
> if we love one another, God abides in us, and His
> love is perfected in us. (1 John 4:8–12)

We are loved by God, and by His grace we love Him,
and through Him we are forever able to love. But, this love
does not change all of our unpleasant circumstances into
more pleasing ones, nor does it change all of the unkind
people into kind and gentle ones; His love changes *us*.

> Love is patient, love is kind, and is not jealous; love
> does not brag and is not arrogant. Does not act
> unbecomingly; it does not seek its own, is not pro-
> voked, does not take into account a wrong suffered.
> Does not rejoice in unrighteousness, but rejoices
> with the truth; bears all things, believes all things,
> hopes all things, endures all things. Love never fails.
> (1 Cor. 13:4–8)

Love builds hope and faith for the journey home. The
earth shifts; life presses in. Circumstances alter events and
people; friends and family disappoint us, betray us or die;
fortunes are lost; disease devastates entire families; accidents happen. And, fear grips our hearts. But, nothing can
separate us from the love of Christ, and "in all these things
we overwhelmingly conquer through Him who loved us."
And, we can know that nothing can separate us from the
love of Christ!

> Who shall separate us from the love of Christ? Shall
> tribulation, or distress, or persecution, or famine,
> or nakedness, or peril, or sword?
>
> Just as it is written, "for thy sake we are being put
> to death all day long; we were considered as sheep
> to be slaughtered."

But in all these things we overwhelmingly conquer through Him who loved us.

For I am convinced that neither death, nor life, nor angels, nor principalities, not things present, nor things to come, nor powers, nor height, nor depth, nor any other created thing, shall be able to separate us from the love of God, which is in Christ Jesus our Lord. (Rom. 8:35–39)

His blood redeems us, and His love restores us. As free agents, we choose to be bondservants of Jesus Christ. We are filled to overflowing with His love. It isn't our love, it is His. And, He gives it without measure. It is a gift which fills and refills us as we pour ourselves into the lives of others. In Him we can be forever loving, because we are forever being loved. Health begins in Him, with loving and being loved.

Whole Foods Instead of "Deceptive Food"

As I recall the dietary regimes which I have followed over the last twenty-five years, I am impressed with the fact that although I followed the conflicting advice of various "experts" in the field of nutrition, each regime improved my health in some measure. I believe that the answer lies in the fact that since 1969 I have eaten whole foods, and not the king's dainties. Absent in every regime were sodas, sugar, white flour, caffeine, packaged and processed foods. Nor did I frequent fast food restaurants which have become an American way of life.

But, it is important to realize that advice which contains only part of the truth is hazardous advice. The Bible offers us dietary guidelines without dangers. Now, the evidence is available. The research studies support God's original diet for man.

My own parents, like many other responsible parents and teachers for the last several decades, depended upon 1) the United States Department of Agriculture guidelines and 2) a medical establishment untrained in health and nutrition as the best providers of information concerning proper diet. The dinner meals which my parents served in our home could have appeared as sample menus in the 1947 edition of the *Childcraft Resource Library*. And, although the breakfasts, lunches, dinners, and desserts were filled with white flour, meat, and dairy products, they would have been considered excellent by the medical and the USDA standards of the day. Until I graduated from high school, my parents, like countless others, issued directives in accordance with the United States Department of Agriculture guidelines: "Do not leave the table until you finish your meat and drink your milk!"

In 1946, the United States Department of Agriculture daily food choices centered around the Basic Seven Food Groups. Here is an ideal diet suggested in *Childcraft, Vol. 10* (1949), based on those Basic Seven: Milk; Meat, including liver and fish; Egg; Whole grain cereal; Tomato or citrus fruits (oranges, grapefruit, tangerines); Green or yellow vegetables; Raw leafy vegetables; and Cod liver oil (or some equally good source of vitamin D).[4]

Then, the USDA abandoned the Basic Seven in favor of the Basic Four Food Groups. However, in the 1972 edition of *Childcraft*, the writers cite the opinions of those nutritionists who base their recommendations on the Basic Seven and those who make recommendations based on the Basic Four.[5] Here is the description of the Basic Four:

1. Milk and milk products, such as cheese and ice cream supply calcium, phosphorus, protein, and riboflavin.

2. Meat, fish, poultry, and eggs supply protein, thiamin, niacin, and mineral elements, such as iron and phosphorus.

3. Vegetables and fruits supply vitamins A and C, iron, thiamin, and certain mineral elements.

4. Breads and cereals, in the whole grain and enriched forms supply thiamin, niacin, riboflavin, and iron as well as protein. Potatoes can be substituted for bread.

In a 1980 health science text, *Keeping Healthy*, published by Laidlaw Brothers, elementary school children were told: "You should eat foods from each group every day. This is a good eating practice. It helps you get all the things you need in foods."[6]

The United States Department of Agriculture presented the information to the textbook publishers and public health officials. Public schools offered these materials as part of their health and science curricula. Parents and students trusted the authority of the textbook publishers and the government schools. Now, the USDA has renounced the old Four Food Groups in favor of the new USA Food Guide Pyramid. And, while the recommendations are a vast improvement over the advice they gave in the forties, fifties, sixties, seventies, and eighties, it is far from the best advice. The 1992 USDA Food Guide Pyramid is in conflict with current research findings. Before 1992, the USDA did not classify one category as more important than another; nor did they warn people about degenerative diseases which result from consuming too much food from certain categories. In the 1992 USDA Food Guide Pyramid, they still did not issue those warnings.

As I began reading health and nutrition books in 1969, I discovered that people had been treating and curing diseases through diet for many years. I also found evidence that contradicted the recommendations made by the U. S. Department of Agriculture. I realized back then that we did not need foods from each of the USDA Basic Four Food Groups. I began to see that the American diet, especially the diet of privileged Americans, featuring expensive cuts of beef, and meat of some sort at every meal, was a diet of death and disease. As I looked back at my recent past, I viewed my college diet and lifestyle with particular horror. On campus or off campus, I enjoyed meals which featured meat, well-cooked vegetables, coffee, tea, and sugary desserts. On social occasions, I consumed alcoholic beverages. Like many people my age, I often stayed up all night studying or just talking. It never occurred to me that premenstrual syndrome, headaches, and occasional bouts of exhaustion had anything to do with an improper diet and sleep deprivation. Much of the time, I experienced tremendous energy and endurance. I performed in numerous stage productions, learned lines quickly and easily, and functioned with little sleep.

I had a glad heart, a tremendous optimism about the future, and a certainty that I would accomplish everything that I wanted most to do. In the sixties, I did not know anything about the relationship between mental attitude and biochemistry. But in light of the research which is now widely reviewed, I believe that my positive attitudes contributed to my good health and to my sense of well-being. I had no knowledge of the reality of Satan and the kingdom of darkness, and I did not believe that the Bible offered anything more than fine literature. And most of all, I knew nothing about the agape love of God. All of my optimism had very shallow roots indeed. I believed that I had found great love and, hence, great meaning in life. But then, the hard times had not yet come.

Many Pathways

Frank had introduced me to a world of food that I hadn't known. He knew the owners of a number of the finest restaurants in the Miami area, many of them Italian. Every Sunday, he cooked for his father and his brother— Sicilian style. When we entertained, Frank cooked, and I assisted. But, he was open to change. We read the same books and reached the same conclusions. The day that we decided to begin our new regime, I bought coffee substitutes, herb tea, herb seasonings, fruits, vegetables and a juicer. I ordered a water distiller. "We'll eat differently," he said, "but when the guests come, I'll cook." And, that is how it worked throughout our marriage. Guests always had options, and they always chose Frank's food. Frank and I ate raw fruits and vegetables, almonds, seeds, and honey. We ate the vegetables in large salads and drank inordinate amounts of carrot juice. I ate a great deal of honey and almonds, reasoning that it was far better than the sugary baked goods I had previously enjoyed. We continued to heed the health enthusiasts who did not recommend eating grain or complex carbohydrates. We seldom ate any cooked food.

The first two weeks on this program, I felt miserable. I experienced such a violent reaction from caffeine and nicotine withdrawal that I would have been too sick to consume either. On two isolated instances, I smoked again. In the first instance, a year from the time that I quit smoking, I smoked an entire package of cigarettes, one after another through the night. And in the other instance, another year later, I smoked a single cigarette. After that, I never smoked again.

Frank and I had complete confidence in our regime. We felt well. In 1970 we decided to buy a second home—a mountain retreat in North Carolina, near Asheville. Frank bought an old army jeep and had it restored, then off we went in February of 1971 to set up our hideaway. The season for the "Gleason Show" had ended, and all of the video taping had been done. We left sunny south Florida and headed into the snow. My father sent his furniture van and workmen ahead to arrange the furniture and install the window treatments. Then my mother and father came for a brief visit. On the afternoon of 14 February, the day after they left, Frank called me to the sofa and whispered, "I'm having a heart attack. Call someone." The man from whom we had purchased our home, Zeb Sheppard, owned a business a few miles away in the Leicester section of Buncombe County where we lived. He was a member of the Emergency Squad. Zeb and another man came within minutes. They carried Frank to the vehicle and had a physician waiting at the hospital. Frank had a myocardial infarction over a previous myocardial infarction. The surgeons installed a temporary pacemaker. Frank spent weeks in intensive care and nearly two months in the hospital. Frank's doctor permitted me to bring Frank freshly extracted carrot juice while he was in intensive care. I bought the juice from a nearby health food store on Wall Street in Asheville.

Frank recovered and elected not to have bypass surgery. He believed that heart disease could be reversed without drugs or surgery. He decided that eating correctly, walking, and leading a simpler life would give him the best hope for getting well. There was no support for that kind of thinking in the medical community at that time. And, no one had done the kind of studies which are now available proving that diet, exercise, and lifestyle changes do in fact reverse heart disease. *Dr. Dean Ornish's Program for Reversing Heart Disease, The Only System Scientifically Proven to Reverse Heart Disease Without Drugs or Surgery* (1990), and Dr. Neal Barnard's *Food for Life* (1993) had not yet been written. And, the Physicians Committee for Responsible Medicine did not yet exist. We had heard about the Shute Clinic in Canada. We had read a book by Dr. Wilfred Shute and believed that vitamin E therapy would be effective in treating Frank's heart disease.[7] We decided to fly to Canada and get our information from the doctors at the Shute Clinic. They discussed the appropriate megadosage of vitamin E and suggested which type of vitamin E to purchase. They offered very little advice concerning diet.

While Frank was in the hospital in Asheville, we sold our home in south Miami—completely furnished. Zeb and Wanda Sheppard and others moved all of our personal effects to Asheville. The possibility of Frank's death had filled me with terror. I did not understand what was happening to me physically. No one explained to me the physiological effects of fear. Suddenly, my body stopped functioning normally. Two years earlier, when I smoked cigarettes, drank coffee, and ate donuts, I felt fine. The symptoms that I developed after Frank's illness plagued me for years thereafter. I suffered from chest pains and shortness of breath; I had never heard of "panic attacks." And, no one I knew in the seventies had ever heard of "panic attacks," not to mention the current phenomenon of "panic attack support groups." I felt dizzy between meals. I felt weak and shaky if I missed meals. I developed migraine headaches, one so severe that the physician had morphine administered to me in the hospital emergency room.

Since the fall of man people have been in danger of being "scared to death." Fear can cause physical discomforts, chronic pain, disease, and death. Only faith in God can reverse the damage done to our bodies by fear.

> For God has not given us a spirit of fear; but of power and love and a sound mind. (2 Tim. 1:17)

> When you lie down, you will not be afraid; When you lie down, your sleep will be sweet. Do not be afraid of sudden fear, Nor of the onslaught of the wicked when it comes; For the Lord will be your confidence, And will keep your foot from being caught. (Prov. 3:24–26)

> He will not fear evil tidings; His heart is steadfast, trusting in the Lord. (Ps. 112:7)

I did not know that I was overcome by fear. I did not connect my physical problems with anxiety. I did not know that I could turn to God for help. When Frank went into surgery to have the temporary pacemaker installed, I went into the chapel and started to pray; then I stopped, suddenly angry. I remember saying to myself, "I don't believe in prayer!" And, I didn't. I did not think anyone could reach the God who might be there, and I did not believe that a personal God could be there at all. I denied my fear and decided to behave as though the absolute best was about to happen. I am sure that I got the idea from my high school drama class. I remembered studying the James Lange theory of emotion. We practiced putting on the "outer cloak of the emotion" in order to portray the inner feeling of the character. This was very different than actually feeling the emotion in order to portray it. I had no other experience or inspiration from which to draw. It seemed to me that I had a role to play. Frank had to know that I believed that he would be fine. That was as close as I could come to actually making things turn out right, to shaping reality. And, in fact, my performance did an amazing amount of good for Frank. He told me later that he knew he would be alright when he saw my face in the intensive care unit. Day by day in the hospital, I appeared to be calm and cheerful. I seemed to others to be fully convinced of Frank's recovery. He became fully convinced as well. I had no conception of life in the Spirit. I did not think that people could truly transcend the circumstances of life. I only understood the determination of my own will. I imagined that I just had a mountain to climb. I didn't know how many mountains were ahead, how treacherous they would be, or that strength of will would never be enough. But, this will not be that story.

By the time the doctor released Frank from the hospital, I had set the house in order. I had collected antiques and old books, and our home looked as though we had lived there for years. When he stepped out of the car, he heard Bach playing at full volume. The sound filled the mountainside. During all of our time there, our lives were filled with music and books and people. And, the people gave us the greatest pleasure of all.

While Frank worked to gain strength, his father and his youngest brother died. He began a struggle with depression that continued until the last six months of his life. Then, we suffered huge financial losses through business and investment failures. We left Asheville in 1972. A few months later while we were living in Coconut Grove, Florida, I discovered that I had had a miscarriage. When the doctor showed me the test results, I was shocked; I had not even realized that I had been pregnant. In 1973, we moved to a small apartment in Ridgewood, New Jersey. Frank appeared to be feeling well, but I did not. I found a health food store in Ridgewood. A woman there talked to me about hypoglycemia. She gave me the name of a physician in New York City who had an excellent reputation for treating hypoglycemia and other diseases. Frank and I both made appointments right away. We had little confidence in our dietary regime. We had even stopped juicing vegetables.

The Best of the Worst Advice and Dietary Regimes

In the seventies the best known treatment for what is called after-meal hypoglycemia was the high-protein/low-carbohydrate diet. A number of well-known doctors who were also authors and speakers advocated this regime. The physician that we visited in New York City gained our confidence. In the waiting room, we met people who testified that their health had vastly improved under his care.

The Regime:

> Morning—Whole Orange, Chicken, Fish, Beef or Lamb, Baked Potato (one half)
>
> Noon—Meat, Poultry, Fish, or Eggs, Green Salad, Baked Potato (or substitute with whole grain bread at one meal)
>
> Night—The same as noon. (Bread only once a day.)
> Also add yellow or green vegetables, cooked or raw.

We went to his office in Manhattan for vitamin shots twice a week. He gave us injections of calcium, B-complex, and B6. He recommended megadoses of vitamins to be taken in tablet or capsule form. Among them were B-complex, vitamins B6, C, E, calcium/magnesium, and a high potency multiple vitamin and mineral supplement.

Both of us felt better on this regime, and my symptoms improved immediately. Since some carbohydrate stimulates insulin, our physician persuaded us that I needed a low-carbohydrate regime to keep the insulin in check. He told us that I had developed hypoglycemia because of the amount of carbohydrates in my diet, especially the fruit and the honey. He suggested the same diet for Frank, but advised that he eat only fish and chicken and avoid red meat. For years, I followed this diet. However, I did best with small, frequent meals; I could not go for long periods of time without food. The dizziness, trembling, weakness, and headaches ceased if I ate small, frequent meals. I felt immeasurably better. This regime differed greatly from our raw foods diet:

Raw Foods Regime

Eat Freely:	Caution:
Raw fruits and vegetables	No meat
Nuts and seeds	No fish
Honey and other natural sweeteners	No poultry
Freshly extracted vegetable juice	No eggs or dairy
	No coffee, tea
	No soft drinks

	Caution:
	No cooked food
	No grain
	No dairy products

High-Protein/Low-Carbohydrate Diet

Eat one portion at each meal:	Caution:
Meat, fish, or poultry	No fruit (except one whole)
Eggs or dairy	No simple sugars (juice, honey, syrup, sweeteners)
Green salad or potatoes	
Other vegetables	

Each Day:	Avoid:
Whole orange for breakfast	Grains and beans
One slice of whole wheat bread	
No coffee; tea at lunch or dinner	
No soft drinks	

This was considered the best advice in 1973. Many doctors in the seventies actually advised their hypoglycemic patients to eat fruit, candy, or even to drink a cola when they felt weak, dizzy, and shaky. Other physicians simply offered no advice at all. Here is what Neal Barnard, M.D., president of the Physicians Committee for Responsible Medicine, says about that type of diet in his book, *Food for Life*, published in 1994:

> The treatment for after-meal hypoglycemia used to be a low carbohydrate diet. Doctors reasoned that since carbohydrate is what stimulates the release of insulin, a low-carbohydrate diet would keep the insulin in check. Some people do feel better on such a diet, but unfortunately, when carbohydrate is taken out of the diet, there are only two things that can go in its place: protein and fat. So the low-carbohydrate approach can lead to far worse problems than it attempts to solve.[8]

But, the Physicians Committee did not exist then. The voices from the medical establishment which we followed in the seventies were the best of the worst advice.

Just before we left the New York City area in 1974, I had yet another physical affliction. We knew that we were about to move, and we had decisions to make. I was finishing an independent study in order to complete my undergraduate degree. Frank had decided to work in television again, but he hadn't found an assignment which interested him. Frank's agent in California called frequently to encourage him to accept one assignment in particular and at the same time to urge us to move to California. As part of my independent project, I wrote a novel in three parts. As I finished writing, I had a sudden realization of my own mortality. I felt consumed with the awareness that life is both fragile and fleeting. Suddenly, the philosophy of the existentialists and the drama of the theater of the absurd flooded my consciousness. I thought of death and, then, nothingness. No reason. No answers. No meaning. The thought of Los Angeles filled me with dread. I visualized

a place out of control with too many cars and too many
people. Frank loved New York City, but he had never
enjoyed living in California. I began awakening each morning at four or five and vomiting. The problem continued
for weeks and grew worse. I could eat very little food. I
went to Manhattan for examinations and x-rays. My weight
dropped below 115. I am 5' 9½", and a size eight hung
loosely. One afternoon, I called my mother to talk about
the writing project. I asked her about death. What did she
think about it and on and on. She listened very quietly.
Then, she said simply, "Terry, you're tired. Perhaps you
and Frank would like to come here for a while." Frank
thought it was a good idea for us to go to Parkersburg
until I got well. "Then, we'll decide what to do," he said.
I never thought that I would want to go back to the Ohio
Valley, but I did want to go back. I wanted to go home.

On the Wings of the Dawn

When I first came home, I could only stay up for a few
hours, and, yet, within several weeks I was on my feet again
and feeling quite normal. Frank and I soon stopped making plans to go to California and began looking at rural
property near Parkersburg. I had lunch a number of times
with a young woman, Prudence Fields, whom I had met
several years earlier. She had grown up in Milwaukee,
graduated from Northwestern University, and appeared in
Funny Girl with Barbara Streisand. We had many things in
common even though our political and social views were
poles apart. Prudence's husband, Bill, had grown up in
Parkersburg. He met Prudence in New York after gradu-
ating from Harvard Law School. Frank and I had spent
several evenings at their home in Marietta, Ohio, during
short visits to Parkersburg to see my family. We had common interests in music and theater and simply enjoyed one
anothers company. I had heard that Prudence had become
a Christian and that she drove around with a Bible on her
dashboard. We met for lunch many times during the summer of 1974. Finally, in September she asked me if I would

like to go to church with her sometime. That was on a Wednesday. I asked her if I could go that night. I hadn't any interest in becoming religious, but I was very interested in visiting with the group of people who had captured her interest. I couldn't imagine that she actually read the Bible for personal guidance. At that time, my consciousness "had been raised" by radical feminism and Marxist socialism.

That Wednesday night, I went to Marietta without Frank. I rode to the church with Prudence and Bill. A prison evangelist ministered that night, and he spoke with exuberance and passion. He presented God's plan for redemption in Christ with love and clarity. I listened intently as he explained that we are born in sin; that we are in need of a Savior; that all have sinned and come short of the glory of God; that we are justified by faith; that faith is a gift of God, not of works, lest any man should boast (Eph. 2:8–9). And, I understood that "with the heart man believes, resulting in righteousness, and with the mouth he confesses, resulting in salvation" (Rom. 10:10). The evangelist spoke of those who promoted a belief in evolutionary theory as people who were at war with God. Then, he quoted God's account of creation in the Book of Genesis. I will never forget saying to myself during his message: "If this is true, then I am wrong about absolutely everything." As people were leaving, I remained in the pew. Prudence told me later that she couldn't imagine why I was sitting there. She did not believe that the sermon could have ministered to me. And yet, there I sat, waiting in the pew. She didn't know what to say to me, and, yet, she knew she had to say something. "Terry, would you like to make profession of faith?" she asked. The question jolted me. I didn't know. And so, I said, "I'd like to pray with your pastor." I knew after the evangelist's message that the words he had spoken were the truth. Only the Holy Spirit could have shown me that. A year later, I discovered Frances Schaeffer. I read the teaching of the Reformation and the sermons of the Great Awakening in America. I found the works of George Whitefield, John Wesley, and Jonathan Edwards. But, that night the Lord changed my heart through the "foolishness of preaching."

> For since in the wisdom of God the world through its wisdom did not come to know God, God was well-pleased through the foolishness of the message preached to save those who believe. (1 Cor. 1:21)

> Because the foolishness of God is wiser than men, and the weakness of God is stronger than men. For consider your calling, brethren, that there were not many wise according to the flesh, not many mighty, not many noble; but God has chosen the foolish things of the world to shame the wise, and God has chosen the weak things of the world to shame the things which are strong, and the base things of the world and the despised, God has chosen, the things that are not, that He might nullify the things that are, that no man should boast before God.

> But by His doing you are in Christ Jesus, who became to us wisdom from God, and righteousness, and sanctification, and redemption, that, just as it is written, "Let him who boasts, boast in the Lord." (1 Cor. 1:25–31)

When I walked into the door that night, Frank was sitting at the dining room table. "Frank, I'm saved!" I said. He looked at me with a blank stare and asked, "From what?" That was in September of 1974. The next day, I began reading the New Testament as fast as I could, one book at a time. I read the Epistle of Paul to the Romans and then the Gospel According to John. Then, I read the rest of the New Testament. In the weeks that followed, Frank listened to the preaching of the Word and read the Bible for himself. On 8 December 1974, Frank asked Christ to touch his heart and to save him. How glorious the view from that wonderful peak and how grateful I felt. But again, I did not know there were mountains to climb and valleys to cross. And again, this is not that story.

I always told Frank that he would live to be very old. We followed our New York doctor's advice. We ate whole foods and never consumed the standard American fare. I realized later that Frank slipped out for an occasional slice of pizza, but I didn't know it back then. We consumed vitamins in megadoses. A local physician gave Frank the same vitamin injections that the doctor in New York had given him. We exercised discipline and did what we thought was best. All of the Christian leaders we knew ate as they pleased and felt that any emphasis on food and health was not of the Lord. By their standards, our diet wasn't wholesome; it was bondage. They believed we ought to have liberty.

Frank died on 30 March 1978 in Lafayette, Louisiana, of a massive heart attack. Surrounded by friends who loved him, the certainty of his eternal peace and joy sustained me. But, in the silence of my home in the weeks that followed, I knew that there was a darkness in my soul.

> Search me, O God, and know my heart; Try me and know my anxious thoughts; And see if there be any hurtful way in me, And lead me in the everlasting way. (Ps. 139:23–24)

Two months after Frank's death, I decided to spend the summer in West Virginia writing about Frank and our life together. I completed the story in two months and laid it aside. During that time, my close friend Polly, in Lafayette, lost her husband quite suddenly after his doctors discovered brain cancer. At the end of the summer, I wanted to rest, to just stop awhile and cancel all that I had planned to do. My parents encouraged me to return to Louisiana to prepare for my general examinations in the fall. They were wise. Romans 8:28–29 consumed my heart and mind. Through those verses my anger and torment left. But, I did not experience the peace that comes with an acceptance of all that God allows. He had not performed that work in my life. I did believe that He had a purpose in every circumstance and that one day I would know it. I would know what it meant to rest in Him. He gave me the strength and the resolve to carry on in spite of my failures.

> And we know that God causes all things to work together for good to those who love God, to those who are called according to His purpose.
>
> For whom He foreknew, He also predestined, to become conformed to the image of His son, that He might be the first-born among many brethren. (Rom. 8:28–29)

Another close friend in Lafayette, Louisiana, Patricia, searched for typists and people who would help me organize mounds of research. In the fall of 1978, I passed my general examinations, and in November of 1978 I left for my second trip to London to do additional research.

Many Christian pastors and teachers experienced an awakening in the city of Lafayette in the seventies, and, after Frank's death, I became acquainted with numerous prayer and Bible study groups all over the city. The Word that I heard preached and taught during the time that I lived in Lafayette took root in my heart and bore fruit in the years ahead.

The Lord surrounded me with kind and capable people in the Department of Speech Communications at Louisiana State University. Under the direction of my major professor, Owen Peterson, I finished my dissertation before the summer of 1979 and received my Ph.D. from Louisiana State University at the end of the summer.

Another Journey

In September of 1979, I began teaching at East Texas Baptist College in Marshall, Texas. That month Gary Dorian flew from Miami to Marshall, and we saw each other for the first time in twelve years. We first met when I was home from college during my spring break in 1966. Gary had come to town to visit a college friend from Parkersburg. I was nineteen, and he was twenty-five. In 1966, he had just signed a recording contract with ABC Paramount Records, and I was finishing my freshman year at Stephens College in Columbia, Missouri. We managed to see each other a number of times in the fall of 1966 and the spring of 1967. In the summer of 1968 I moved to Boca Raton, Florida, and Gary lived in Manhattan. During the summer of 1968, we stopped corresponding. In December of 1968, Gary married a girl he met in New York who had been his sister's roommate. Our lives went in directions which neither of us had planned or imagined.

Gary continued in the music business. He wrote and produced jingles and filmscores in New York. He also performed for a number of years as the lead singer for the B. J. Thomas Band and served as the band's director. Gary left New York in 1976 after separating from his wife. Their marriage ended in divorce on 30 March 1978. Gary's two daughters were nine and six years old at the time.

Gary heard about Frank's death in the spring of 1978 and called my parents in August of 1978 to get my telephone number. I then wrote to him about my life in Christ and my work at the university. In September 1979, he asked if he could visit me in Marshall. I agreed, and he flew to the nearest airport in Shreveport, Louisiana. He returned for a visit in October. Then, I flew to Miami for a weekend in October. We were married in Lafayette, Louisiana, on 9 November 1979.

Not only had my grieving process for Frank not ended, it had not even begun. Grieving requires rebuilding; it is a deep work. It is most of all an acceptance of suffering when our flesh desires personal peace and happiness. Grief is essential. And through it, God takes our anxious thoughts and hurtful ways and leads us into His everlasting way (Ps. 139:23–24). But, the flesh must die.

In the first two years of marriage to Gary, I learned that the death of a spouse is not the greatest sorrow of life. And, at age forty-seven, I am certain that I have not known the greatest sorrows of life. However, I felt the greatest turmoil and anguish I had ever known when I realized that being happily married to Gary, or even remaining married to Gary, required more than my determination. It came as a great surprise to me that he didn't think my queer ways of eating were wonderful, and that he didn't think my inability to cook was tolerable. Nothing in life or literature had prepared me for such incompatibility. I didn't find anything wrong with him, and I was absolutely shocked that he didn't find me perfectly delightful. And, delighted he was not. Gary had made a profession of faith in October before we were married. He saw the truth of God's Word, and he embraced it. But, there were strongholds, in the spirit and in the flesh. He had begun smoking marijuana when he worked in the music business. Although he quit using the drug when we were married, by December of that year, he was using it again. I could not understand the bondage, and I did not know his agony until months later.

If Frank and I moved like birds on the wing, Gary and I collided like ships in the night. He wept before God, but I did not know it. He lived in despair, but I couldn't see. My love smothered him; my cheerfulness exasperated him; my desire for children panicked him; my strong will angered him. But, God gave me a faith that truly transcended our circumstances. Even when I felt defeat and waves of hopelessness, I remembered God's faithfulness. I believed— by the power of God's Spirit—that Gary wanted to walk with God and that he would. But, I had not planned to suffer! I had just fallen wonderfully in love and stepped off the edge of the earth into marriage so that I could quit grieving as a widow. In this marriage, I found something harder than grief.

I had seen in Gary the gentle man I had known him to be when we first met in 1966. I believed that the changes were a lie, and that God would make a way. Without revealing his desperation, Gary moved through the obligations and responsibilities of his life in quiet desperation. When he smoked marijuana, he did so alone, by our pool or in front of an open window. We sold our home in Coral Gables and moved to Homestead, Florida. I quit teaching at the University of Miami. I believed then, as I do now, that God called me to be a worker at home, to learn from Him how to walk in obedience to Titus 2:4-5. I have been "home" ever since.

Then, in January 1982, after parting dozens of times during 1980 and 1981, Gary quietly asked me to take everything and leave. We had placed most of our furniture in storage. We had moved into a small duplex in Homestead. With tears running down our faces, we said, "I love you." And off I went, back to Louisiana, leaving Gary with his clothing, a radio, and his Bible. That night Gary cried out before the Lord. And, although I did not know about it until ten days later, Gary had a Damascus Road experience that night. He asked God to deliver him and set him free. He fell asleep on the floor, weeping before the Lord. When he awoke he knew that God had indeed touched him and that he had been set free. He never used, nor desired, an intoxicant from that moment on. When he called ten days later, my spirit bore witness to the Spirit in him. God laid the foundation for our marriage on the ashes of our dreams.

On the drive from Homestead, Florida, to Lafayette, Louisiana, I had a revelation from God the same day that Gary cried out to Him. I knew that the Lord could make a way and enlarge the steps beneath my feet (Ps. 18:36). I knew that in Him I could serve Him and enjoy Him whether my marriage blossomed or failed. But, I didn't believe I could simply marry again and go on. I thought about never having children, about living apart from Gary for years while God did a work in his life. Could God enable me to walk in love, joy, peace, patience, kindness, goodness, faithfulness, gentleness, and self-control as I trusted God to work in His own time and in His own way? On that long drive, I heard the answer. Yes, He could enable me to do that, but I needed deliverance. All of those months I had wanted Gary to walk in Christ for me, to end my pain. By the time that I arrived in Lafayette, God had shown me the work to be done in me. And, in my heart I answered: I love the Lord, because He hears my voice and my supplications. Because He has inclined His ear to me, therefore I shall call upon Him as long as I live (Ps. 116:1-2).

Without His mercy I would have reaped what I had sown.

> So they shall eat of the fruit of their own way, And be satiated with their own devices. For the waywardness of the naive shall kill them, And the complacency of fools shall destroy them. But he who listens to me shall live securely, And shall be at ease from the dread of evil. (Prov. 1:31-33)

I had the assurance of His Word that He would complete the work that He had begun in Gary and the work that He had begun in me.

> For I am confident of this very thing, that He who began a good work in you will perfect it until the day of Christ Jesus. (Phil. 1:6)

During those first two years of marriage, God revealed His power, His mercy, and His faithfulness. In the middle of all of the turmoil, we had two wonderful summers with Gary's daughters, Kim and Stacey, in 1980 and 1981, and a delightful Christmas with them in 1981 in Parkersburg, West Virginia. Kim was age eleven and Stacey age eight the summer of 1980. They made professions of faith that summer in our home.

Whatever struggles Gary and I faced, nothing interfered with our enjoyment of the children. Gary committed himself to making his time with them both rich and meaningful. I remember looking into their faces and saying that when people know Christ they have the power to be married forever. It came as a response to one of their questions that first summer in Coral Gables. I thought about my answer again and again and again. I don't believe I could ever have given up on Gary or ever have stopped waiting for God to touch our lives, not with their faces before me. Loving them through Him transformed my life.

In February 1982, Gary and I wanted to know whether or not we would be able to conceive a child. We sought medical advice. After several months, we discovered that we were both infertile. That spring my father asked Gary to manage one of his businesses in Parkersburg. We moved to West Virginia in May. In July, we went before the elders of the church and asked them to anoint us with oil. We asked the Lord to give us a child. We conceived our daughter, Jessica, that same month. She was born 10 April 1983; our second child, Canaan, was born on 29 August 1984. God heals.

The Worst of the Best Advice and Dietary Regimes

If the High-Protein/Low-Carbohydrate Diet is the best of the worst dietary regimes; then the Macrobiotic Diet is the worst of the best regimes. I say that it is among the best regimes because it features intact grains as the basis for a healthful diet. Complex carbohydrates are a critical feature in the macrobiotic regime. I came to realize, to my delight, that by eating grains, vegetables, and beans I allowed my body to gradually absorb glucose; consequently, my body did not respond with jolts of insulin. Raw food regimes which do not include a significant quantity of intact grain and a small amount of cooked vegetables create stress on the body. They are not balanced. The macrobiotics also caution against having much raw fruit. While large quantities of raw fruit are life-giving for some people, many people cannot handle the rapid rush of simple sugar which even whole fruits give them. I have counseled many overweight women who have not been able to regain strength or to lose weight until they have eliminated all simple sugars, even fruits, from their diets.

In 1982, I began reading everything that I could find concerning diet during pregnancy. And, once again, I braced myself for the contradictory advice concerning the best foods. As a Christian, I found the spiritual roots of the macrobiotic regime to be more than a little troublesome. Michio Kushi's teaching and his *Universal Way of Health and Happiness* are not derived from a revelation of God's Word.[9] However, the self-reflections that he advocates are counterfeits of actual biblical imperatives. Michio Kushi's questions reveal a certain respectfulness and gentleness:

1. Did I eat properly today, and did I chew well?

2. Did I think of my parents and elders today, with love and respect?

3. Did I happily greet everyone today?

4. Did I marvel today at the wonders of nature?

5. Did I thank everyone and appreciate whatever I experienced today?

In macrobiotic philosophy, there is a shadow of the truth. But as Christians, we find in the fullness of God's Word the Truth which enables us to walk in His everlasting way. In the preceding five reflections, man seeks to have a pure heart. In contrast, the following principles express a reliance on God's Word.

1. Did I eat the whole foods which God has provided or did I eat "deceptive food" which brings about disease? (Prov. 23:1–3)

Did my choices regarding food and every other area of my life bring honor and glory to God? (1 Cor. 10:31)

2. Did I honor my parents?

"Honor your father and your mother that your days may be prolonged in the land which the Lord your God gives you." (Exod. 20:12)

And did I (as a man) seek out the wisdom of older men who are "temperate, dignified, sensible, sound in faith, in love, in perseverance"? (Titus 2:2)

And did I (as a woman) seek out the women who are "reverent in their behavior, not malicious gossips, nor enslaved to much wine, teaching what is good that they may encourage the younger women to love their husbands, to love their children, to be sensible, pure, workers at home, kind, being subject to their own husbands, that the word of God may not be dishonored"? (Titus 2:3)

3. Did I "rejoice in the Lord" in all that I thought and all that I did today? And did I let my "forbearing spirit be known to all men"? (Phil. 4:4-5)

4. Did I marvel at the Lord's care over all His works? (Ps. 104:1-35)

5. Did I express gratitude for everyone and everything in my life this day?

But we request of you, brethren, that you appreciate those who diligently labor among you, and have charge over you in the Lord and give you instruction.

And that you esteem them very highly in love because of their work. Live in peace with one another.

And we urge you brethren, admonish the unruly, encourage the fainthearted, help the weak, be patient with all men.

See that no one repays evil for evil, but always seek after that which is good for one another and for all men.

Rejoice always; pray without ceasing; in everything give thanks; for this is God's will for you in Christ Jesus. (1 Thess. 5:12-18)

Many Christian brothers and sisters are walking in bondage to food. Their appetites control their lives. Craving unwholesome food is only one undesirable appetite, but it is one which we must acknowledge.

For many walk, of whom I often told you, and now tell you even weeping, that they are enemies of the cross of Christ, whose God is their appetite, and whose glory is in their shame, who set their minds on earthly things. (Phil. 3:18-19)

For those who are according to the flesh set their minds on the things of the flesh, but those who are according to the Spirit, the things of the Spirit. (Rom. 8:5)

Eating is a spiritual matter! We are not our own. We were bought with a price. If people who do not know Christ can walk in discipline and self-control, surely we as Christians can walk free from bondage to food.

I took what I found to be helpful from the macrobiotic dietary regime. Eating an abundance of complex carbohydrates for the first time in my life greatly improved my strength and stamina. I ate substantially less fat and protein and many, many times more complex carbohydrates. But, during that period I probably placed too much emphasis on combining foods such as grains and beans in order to get all eight essential amino acids at one meal. Now, it is widely known that food-combining is not necessary to obtain sufficient protein from a vegetarian diet if we eat a good supply of grains and vegetables. I had relied on early editions of Frances Moore Lappe's book, *Diet for a Small Planet,* and other resources.

The misinformation regarding the amount of protein our body requires still abounds. In the eighties, throughout the time that I gave birth to the children and nursed them, I served fish and chicken. We also had meatless meals several evenings a week; but those meals always had both grain and beans or grain and tofu. I heeded the advice of those who recommended including all of the essential amino acids during the same meal. Although I knew that we did not need to eat meat, dairy, and eggs, I did not know that even my meatless meals can provide far more protein than our bodies require. The children drank soy milk. And to meet our B12 requirement, we ate miso soup regularly. This vitamin is produced by bacteria and other one-celled organisms. Miso is processed from soybeans and cereal grains such as barley, rice, and wheat, with sea salt, through slow fermentation. I am grateful for the knowledge about food which I gleaned from macrobiotic teachings. As a Christian, I appreciate the encouragement from macrobiotic writers regarding an appropriate attitude toward meal planning and meal preparation. The Holy Spirit birthed a desire in me to learn and to love the tasks which are essential in providing nourishing food for friends and family. If we as Christians imitate the ways of the world in regard to "getting out of the kitchen" and "eating on the run," then we cannot hope to enjoy the healing and health benefits of food and fellowship. Nurturing and serving one another are His way. If we seek to escape those joys, we are deceived.

Finding the Path

Switching the emphasis of our diet from high-protein/low-carbohydrate to a diet high in complex carbohydrates, particularly grains, greatly benefited our health. I experienced an increase in my stamina and a more stable blood sugar level. I was able to eat less frequently. Although we greatly reduced our protein intake, we did not consume the low protein diet which we now enjoy. The truth concerning the amount of protein our bodies need is now widely published as a result of the sheer weight of scientific evidence. The average American consumes three to five times the amount of protein (over one hundred grams) than is necessary for optimal health. Major commercial industries profit from a population convinced they must eat over one hundred grams of protein per day. But, at last the news is out. Numerous studies reveal that high-protein diets cause degenerative disease: cancer, gout, arthritis, osteoporosis—the list goes on. In Part Two, we discuss the ease with which we meet our protein requirement by consuming the foods which provide optimal health and healing.

Not only did I benefit by eating less protein and more complex carbohydrates, I experienced the enormous health benefits of the increased hormonal activity stimulated by pregnancy and lactation. I gave birth to my first child at the age of thirty-six and my second child at the age of thirty-seven. I nursed Jessica for three years, and Canaan for two years. Thankfulness and joy filled my heart. I embraced the call on my life with gratitude because I knew that God had answered prayer. The Lord had given me my heart's desire, and I had the maturity to apprehend the wonder of it all. The gladness in my heart surely strengthened my body as well. A mother can physically feel the blessing of God as she nurses her baby. During that time of bonding, both the mother and the baby profit in this loving exchange. I also nursed my other two children—Christian for nine months, and Jenna for two years.

God blessed us with healthy pregnancies, vaginal deliveries, and healthy babies. And, for the first time since I was twenty-four years old, I could eat anything. I didn't react adversely to simple sugars, and I didn't feel weak and shaky when I missed meals. Apart from the usual discomforts of pregnancy, I enjoyed abundant health.

On 26 April 1987, our son Christian was born. During that pregnancy, Gary and I wrote two Christian musicals. I required less sleep. At night I read the Word and wrote lyrics. Then, in October of 1987, when Christian was six months old, my father discovered that he had cancer. On the flight to Rochester, Minnesota, I held Christian on my lap and read Frank Peretti's novel, *This Present Darkness*. Peretti's insights were God's provision for that trial. I thought of my father's strength and generosity and his desire to help each of his children in every way possible. His words and deeds promoted enormous good will among his children and their spouses. But, in spite of his boundless generosity toward me, we often clashed. Dad had a strong will and a strong personality. We disagreed about many issues. Dad did not share my faith in Christ. But, in spite of our different values and convictions, I had always longed for his approval and acceptance. During that flight, for the first time in my life, I saw my father's need, and not my own. I considered his struggles, turmoil, and unrest without Christ. I wanted him to walk in health and happiness. But, most of all I wanted him to walk with God for all eternity. My plane landed just after Dad was scheduled to go into surgery. But, there was a delay, and we had time together before his operation.

People of any age do not simply rush to the feet of Christ because they are sick and dying. Whenever that awakening comes, it comes by the power of the Holy Spirit. I had spoken to my father about the Lord many, many times since that September in 1974 when I came to Christ. My faith put a certain wedge between us, which we constantly worked through and around. But, as we sat together on his bed at Saint Marys (*sic*) Hospital in October of 1987, he opened his heart to me and to the Lord. He spoke with humility, tenderness, and candor. He knew that he might not live through surgery and that if he did live, he mightn't live for very long. We prayed and discussed the Word of God and prayed again. And, from that time until his death nearly two years later, I knew, beyond a shadow of a doubt, that Dad had received new life in Christ. "The old things passed away," and all of his ways, in spite of his illness, became new (1 Cor. 5:17). Dad and I talked heart-to-heart until he died. But, this intermission is more than bearable. I will be with him for all eternity.

Dad fought as hard as he could to live. He had access to what he believed to be the best medical advice that money can buy. It never occurred to me to seek or to discuss alternative cancer treatment. Dad had every confidence that traditional medicine offered him the best hope for recovery. For years, Dad had regarded my own dietary regimes as eccentric and somewhat annoying. I had no credibility as a cancer expert. Had those whom he considered to be America's best and brightest physicians offered him a radical diet and nutritional therapy as an answer to curing cancer, he would have heeded their advice. But, no one in the mainstream medical establishment offered him an alternative to chemotherapy and radiation. Doctors advised him to eat whatever he could get down. With every chemotherapy and radiation treatment, his health deteriorated. He could eat very little and eventually he could not taste the food he ate. I was with my father daily in the hospital and at home during the last six weeks of his life.

He would have considered no regime too strict, no diet too confining, if he could have had his life in exchange for the license to eat as he pleased.

But, disease and death had no victory. Dad depended on prayer, and he knew that he belonged to God. We prayed together almost every day during the thirty months of his illness. I lived in Florida, and much of our time together was on the telephone. A precious pastor and friend visited Dad every day for months before he died. He stood with my brothers, my mother, my sister, and me as Dad went home one Sunday morning in June of 1989. We sang together as we stood by his bed. Every death in Christ is a victory.

In August of 1990, Gary and I and the four children moved to Rock Hill, South Carolina. Gary accepted a position operating two of our family's motels in the Carolinas. During my father's illness, my mother and younger brother managed all of Dad's business interests. Tending to Dad and taking care of the businesses proved to be difficult. At the time of my father's death the businesses presented numerous challenges. My mother, my siblings, and I were committed to each other and to keeping harmony in the family, but we did not share a common view regarding the numerous crises.

In May 1991, Gary and I and the children drove to Boulder, Colorado, for the wedding of Gary's daughter, Stacey. The children were attendants for their sister. Gary composed and performed a song for Stacey and her husband, Pat. Stacey and Pat are committed Christians, and today they minister to the youth at Faith Baptist Chapel North in Broomfield, Colorado.

When we returned to South Carolina, Gary decided that he needed to resign from the family business in the interest of building family relationships and preserving family unity. I had learned, once again, that death is not the greatest sorrow. Conflicts and misunderstandings with those we love create turmoil and a burning sense of loss. In the absence of Dad's leadership, it seemed to me at one point that we were truly lost as a family; that we hadn't simply lost Dad, but that my mother, my brothers, my sister, and I had lost each other as well. But, in spite of the strains of adversity, God protected and preserved the natural affection which we have felt for one another since childhood. Mother's love pricked our hearts. It has been the pattern of her life to meet the needs of others, to walk in self-denial and self-control, and to love her children unconditionally. Her life continues to serve us as a reservoir of kindness and mercy.

Just before we moved to Rock Hill in August of 1990, I quit nursing Jenna who had just turned two. I wore a size twelve dress, and I expected to return to my normal size just as I had with the other children. But, by May of 1991, I wore a size eighteen dress. I had not changed our whole foods regime in any way. But, my body had changed. I never expected to be overweight. I thought that by eating "good foods" always and "junk food" never, I would never have a weight problem. I scheduled a routine physical, and the physician told me that I was simply getting older, that I needed to exercise more and eat less. When I told him the kinds of foods that I ate and explained my regime, he said that I must be eating more than I realized. He suggested that I keep a journal and write down everything that I ate. He was sure that I would discover that I was eating more than I thought. I winced. I had read articles written by specialists who design weight and eating disorder programs. Overweight people underestimate their intake by 40 percent each day; lean people, by 20 percent. His advice was to count calories and to limit my food intake. And, although I did not have the answer to my problem, I knew that he did not have the answers either.

During that period, I did not recognize two important factors which are essential if we are to maintain good health in the middle of challenging circumstances. First, I did not consider the direct relationship between mental attitude and biochemistry, although I knew that the Word of God warns us that there is such a connection.

My son, give attention to my words; Incline your
ear to my sayings. Do not let them depart from
your sight; Keep them in the midst of your heart.
For they are life to those who find them, And health
to all their whole body. (Prov. 4:20-22)

Pleasant words are as honeycomb, sweet to the soul,
and health to the bones. (Prov. 16:24)

I create the fruit of the lips; Peace, peace to him
that is far off, and to him that is near, saith the
Lord; and I will heal him. (Isa. 57:19)

I believe that by responding with anger and fear to the
circumstances concerning the family businesses and circumstances beyond my control, I poisoned my own body.
Scientific studies reveal that all of our thoughts and emotions eventually impact the hormonal system—often with
the power to create disease or to end it.[10] When we delay
our resolve to walk in peace and forgiveness, we pay a
price.

Secondly, I did not understand which foods are the
most effective in strengthening the body and preventing
disease. And, while I focused on whole foods, foods that
had not been processed and devitalized, I neglected to
investigate and to choose foods which would build optimal
health. All of us, at various times, need a nutritional boost
to meet the demands placed on our bodies. We need to
consume the "power foods." And, in Part Two we'll discuss
what they are. With the "power foods," we can eat our way
thin and strong.

Gary and I and the children were blessed with precious
friends, and we enjoyed an excellent homeschool support
group in Rock Hill. Through a good friend, we discovered
the advantages of freshly milled flour over the sacks of
organic whole wheat which I purchased from the health
store or natural foods cooperative. At first, I made bread
by hand and milled the wheat berries in my blender. At the
time of Stacey's wedding, we stayed with friends in Fort
Collins, Colorado, who gave Gary an autobakery for his
birthday. One simple machine kneaded the dough and

baked the bread. At that time in our lives, such a machine made breadmaking enticing.

In October of 1991, we moved to upstate South Carolina. We sold our home in Rock Hill and bought a home in Landrum, thirty miles from Greenville. We pursued our interests in home food systems, particularly grain mills and advanced food dehydration machines. Having discovered the health benefits of freshly milled flour and the high nutritional value of dehydrated foods, we sought information from the leading manufacturers of grain mills and food dehydrators. We knew that numbers of people were interested in learning how to eat simply and healthfully and in getting "back to basics." We sought out special interest periodicals which reached those groups: home-education magazines and newsletters, survival catalogues and newsletters, and macrobiotic magazines and supply catalogues. Through those resources, we located authors who had written unbiased evaluations of kitchen specialty equipment and who offered advice in choosing home food systems. Three state-of-the-art machines changed our lives— a grain mill, an advanced food dehydrator, and, eventually, the world standard breadmaker mixer. Grinding wheat for flour and flaking grain for cereals gave us a tremendous nutritional advantage.

Gary and I developed an enthusiasm about the machines, our new household servants. They enabled us to provide wholesome foods in a short amount of time and with very little effort. Bread is a staple for most families. And, bread made from freshly milled flour is the only health-building bread that exists. Ninety percent of the nutritional value of the wheat berry is contained in the wheat germ and wheat germ oil. All of the essential vitamins oxidize within three days from the time the berry is ground into flour. Hence the wheat germ and wheat germ oil cannot be left in commercial baked goods. According to Dr. Wilfred Shute, a pioneer in the research of vitamin E, the lack of vitamin E in the American diet can be traced back to the beginning of commercial milling which eliminated the wheat germ from the flour. Wheat germ is a significant source of vitamin E, a vital nutrient. If the wheat germ remained, rancidity, mold, and spoilage would ruin the products before the baked goods reached the consumer. Consequently, baked goods made from commercial flour lack the delicious flavor which characterizes bread made from freshly milled flour.

Gary and I realized that we had a message and a mission. We knew that making delicious bread from freshly milled flour could be an inviting first step to better health for many people. That excitement gave birth to a home business. We thought of numerous ways to market the machines we enjoyed, and we began writing technical reports and product presentation brochures. We made thousands of small efforts and eventually a buyer for a chain of stores gave us a purchase order for a large number of dehydrators. In November of 1992, the company flew us to Salt Lake City, and Gary and I agreed to operate a Corporate East Office out of our home. We worked in that capacity from November 1992 until September 1993. In the fall of 1993, a new company, Nutriflex, expanded the Magic Mill product line and began distributing their products directly to the consumer through network marketing.

As a result of our involvement with Magic Mill, we were immersed in nutritional research and customer relations. We answered a toll-free information number which put us in touch with people all over the country. People called not just to ask about milling, baking, and dehydrating. They asked for nutritional counseling as well. Many people had children who suffered from food allergies. Others seemed to be sensitive to various foods. Many parents and children couldn't tolerate the wheat in commercial baked goods. Often women called who were sick and tired, and they wanted to do whatever was necessary in order to feel better. They wanted to know how to plan better meals for families. We recommended books, newsletters, and various other resources. Eventually, these hundreds and hundreds of conversations lead us to write an

Eating Better Resource Guide and Video Seminar for the company.[11] And, we saw again and again that milling and baking were the giant first steps to better health for most households. During the winter of 1992, in Landrum, we came to realize that many families consume a diet of devitalized, chemically laden, saturated fat-filled food without realizing that those habits lead only to disease.

In the spring of 1992, I began to feel increasingly tired every day. "Lord," I asked repeatedly, "why am I feeling tired, and why am I overweight?" I had seen people flourish when they began eating exactly as I ate. Our dietary regime conformed to the guidelines established by the USDA Food Guide Pyramid. Not only did we use whole grains as the foundation; all of our flour products—bread, muffins, rolls, pizza, cookies, crackers—were made from freshly milled flour. In addition to those foods, I served predominantly intact grains for lunch and dinner. We ate a variety of raw fruits and vegetables. When I cooked, I used stainless steel, waterless cookware. We ate beans or tofu perhaps once a day. We skinned our chicken and ate steamed or baked chicken and fish several times a week. With high-fiber pancakes and baked goods made from freshly milled flour, we ate honey, grain sweeteners, and sugarless fruit spreads. We limited our intake of dairy to the mozzarella cheese we used on pizza. We prepared only whole foods. And, although Gary and the children ate whatever foods were served to them at church dinners or at the homes of friends, I remained careful to avoid all sugar, products made with white flour, and monosodium glutamate. In spite of all that I did to insure that I ate a wholesome, "balanced" diet, I began to experience fatigue throughout most of the day. I read about the health benefits of green tea and reasoned that the small amount of caffeine that it contained wouldn't bother me. The Japanese had enjoyed the health benefits of green tea for years. I began drinking only a few cups; soon after, I made a pot in the morning and another pot later in the day. In May 1992, I "crashed." While driving down the highway, I had

a serious hypoglycemic episode. I got off the road and
managed to get food into my body just in time. The next
few days after that episode were a nightmare. I felt as
badly as I had in my twenties when I first suffered from
hypoglycemia. But, I was not in my twenties. I was forty-
five years old, fifty pounds overweight, and the symptoms
which I experienced terrified me. In his book, *Food for Life*,
Dr. Neal Barnard states that hypoglycemic symptoms include "headache, poor concentration, fatigue, confusion,
palpitations, anxiety, sweating, and tremulousness."[12] And,
he explains that the symptoms are caused by "the brain
not getting the glucose it needs, and also, by adrenaline
and related hormones becoming more active when the
blood sugar falls."[13] Panic increases the problem. And, I
experienced panic!

Then, after the second week of the nightmare, I cried
out to the Lord for specific guidance. "What, Lord, am I
to eat, and what am I to do?" I thought of Daniel who
sought permission from the commander of the officials to
be given only vegetables to eat and water to drink that he
might not defile himself (Dan. 1:8–14).

> And at the end of ten days their [Daniel,
> Hananiah, Mishael, and Azariah] appearance
> seemed better and they were fatter than all of the
> youths who had been eating the king's choice
> food. So the overseer continued to withhold their
> choice food and the wine they were to drink, and
> kept giving them vegetables. (Dan. 1:15–16)

I had an uneasiness at that time, in spite of Daniel,
chapter one and Genesis 1:29, about ever going on an all-
vegetarian diet. The Lord meets us where we are. I asked
him to show me how to restore my health.

I ate vegetables, lightly cooked, and large bowls of raw
vegetables and steamed brown rice. I used extra virgin
olive oil in liberal amounts and some sea salt on nearly
everything. I ate a can of red salmon (or occasionally
sardines) every day as a source of omega 3 fatty acids. I ate
no fruit and no simple sugars of any kind (no honey, grain

sweeteners, or fruit sweeteners). I ate only extra virgin olive oil, no other oil. I stopped drinking green tea, and, within a few months, I even stopped drinking herb tea. I only drank water. At first, I awoke in the very early morning, ate, and went back to bed. Gradually, I was able to increase the length of time between meals. A typical raw vegetable lunch would include a large bowl filled with cabbage, carrots, yellow squash, purple onions, cauliflower, and garbanzo beans. I cooked broccoli lightly (crunchy and bright green) and stirred it in last. I added salmon, extra virgin olive oil, and sea salt.

Within two weeks, I was stable. We traveled to Springfield, Missouri, for my stepdaughter Kim's graduation and wedding. Both Kim and her fiancé, Darren Lancaster, graduated from Baptist Bible College on the same weekend that they were married. All of us were in the wedding. Gary composed and performed a song for them. The children were attendants, and I read a passage of Scripture. The Lancasters moved to Dallas, Texas, where they now serve the Lord at Creekside Community Church. When we returned to South Carolina, I continued to feel very well.

By the summer of 1993, I had been feeling very well for a year. I wore a size twelve dress. I began writing the *Eating Better Program Guide and Video Seminar* for Magic Mill/Nutriflex. We studied the benefits of various beans and grains and experimented with ways in which to prepare them. I located information written by a group of physicians in England which discussed the ways to determine and eliminate food intolerances. We had so many requests for information about food allergies and food intolerances that we continually searched for information that would help people to resolve those problems. That summer, I discovered the incredible grain spelt. I personally experienced the ways in which this grain is better tolerated by the body than any other grain. I felt energized after eating it. The grain sustained me for many hours longer than brown rice or millet. Spelt is not only high in carbohydrates, it also has all eight essential amino acids.

There is more crude fiber in spelt than in wheat, and the grain is high in B-vitamins. Also, this grain has a number of immune-stimulating properties. For me, it has been a rejuvenator. In the summer of 1993, I replaced my daily portions of steamed organic short grain brown rice with spelt. Having had rice regularly for nearly a decade, I reasoned that I would do well to omit it for a while.

Then, I decided to omit potatoes from my regime. As I studied various elimination diets prepared by those who treat food intolerances, I noticed that potatoes appeared on several lists. Like most people, I had eaten potatoes regularly for a number of years. The occasional, baffling fatigue that I had experienced after meals during my wonderful year of recovery ended. With those two simple changes, adding spelt and dropping potatoes, my stamina continued to increase. By September of 1993, I wore a size ten dress.

I did not lose weight and gain vitality by going on an exercise program, although I led a physically active life. I ate my way thin by consuming large bowls of vegetables and grain. I did not—ever once—count, or consider, calories or fat grams. I believe that the foods that I ate are foods which are essential for optimal health. I did not have all the answers then, and I don't now. But, the answers which I did have, changed my life. As I ate "power foods," I gained strength and lost excess weight. Although I did not count fat grams, I ate only the fat found in beans and grains, salmon, sardines, and extra virgin olive oil. Although I have since omitted the fish, for reasons which I will discuss later, the truth is that I lost weight and regained my strength by eating daily "high-fat" salmon, rich in omega 3 fatty acids.

One affliction plagued me off and on during that triumphant two-year revitalization period. Sometimes, after working particularly hard, or for no reason I could imagine, I experienced pharyngeal spasms. I went to the emergency room on one occasion. Then, after another incident in the winter of 1994, I called a Christian friend who is a physician. He thought that the spasms were related to the stress of a demanding work schedule. He suggested that I take a tranquilizer to alleviate the problem. I couldn't accept that remedy. In the summer of 1994, after returning from a trip to West Virginia with the children, I sought the Lord for a specific solution. I didn't know what I could do—except pray. When I felt my throat tightening, I attempted to get very still, and I began to meditate on the Word. His Word gave me peace as the episodes passed. Still, I asked God for deliverance.

I could think of no changes I needed to make regarding the foods I consumed. Also, I consumed a variety of isolated vitamins and minerals in the form of nutritional supplements. And, although numbers of people had given me information about whole foods concentrates, I had little interest in reading the materials. The number and variety of health claims made by those selling the products seemed too fantastic to be credible. For years, I had been taught to use specific vitamins and minerals to alleviate specific nutritional deficiencies. I had every confidence that finding the necessary vitamins and minerals in sufficient potency could solve most health problems. Whole foods concentrates seemed to me to be nutritionally weak compared to the megavitamins I had been accustomed to taking. Then, in July of 1994, I began reading literature about green barley juice. What I discovered surprised me. The nutrients in this whole-food concentrate work at the cellular level, giving the body the essential nutrients which each cell needs. Instead of targeting symptoms, as drugs do, the vitamins, minerals, enzymes, protein, and chlorophyll, which are present in the green barley juice, work at the cellular level and enable the body to fight all disease. The healthy cells enable the body to heal itself. Healing takes place seemingly regardless of the disease. People taking the green barley juice discover that their bodies heal themselves of heart disease, hepatitis, asthma, obesity, constipation, cancer, skin diseases, acne, and on and on.[14] The testimonies are staggering!

I had been unwilling to really listen and to learn. If illnesses are induced by an imbalance of minerals, enzymes, and vitamins, then the concentrated nutrients in this whole-food concentrate could break the vicious cycle and enable the body to heal itself. Since the very first day that I began taking the green barley juice, I have not had a single pharyngeal spasm. I praise God for His mercy and His provision. He leads and directs us. He answers prayer.

In August 1994, I met Dr. Mary Ruth Swope, Christian author, speaker, and nutritionist. We spent time together as house guests at the home of a mutual friend. I literally sat at her feet listening to her spiritual insights as well as her knowledge about nutrition. Her calling is to warn the body of Christ about the ways in which consuming "deceptive food" is causing many to perish. As I discussed my regime and told her the ways in which God lead me to optimal health and weight, she understood it all. But, she made one suggestion: go the way of the Genesis 1:29 diet. Avoid fish altogether and use organic flax seed oil as your source of omega 3 fatty acids. Dr. Swope indicated that research shows that all marine life has been contaminated by pollutants.

The Physicians Committee for Responsible Medicine shares this view about fish. In addition to the contamination problem, which I discuss later, fish contain cholesterol and fat, including saturated fat. Now that man has contaminated the environment, fish are filled with pesticides and chemical pollutants of all kinds. Pollutants in our rivers, streams, and oceans make it hazardous to eat fish. Since August of 1994, I have taken Dr. Swope's advice.

In September of 1994, Gary and I met Rev. George Malkmus who was healed of colon cancer and numerous other physical problems after changing to a natural diet and lifestyle in 1976. We believe that his message to the body of Christ has the anointing of God. As we heard him speak for the first time, Gary kept nudging me and nodding his head. As we spoke to Rev. Malkmus and his wife, Rhonda, we were blessed by the testimonies of numerous people who have been healed by changing their diet. God has truly provided food as His first provision for healing and health. When we got home, Gary got the Champion Juicer out from under the counter; it has been in use ever since. Certainly, no one needed a juice extractor in the Garden of Eden. But, our bodies are now weakened by food products and environmental hazards which did not exist even a century ago. Now, as I look at the produce, mainly carrots, stacked up in our backup refrigerator in the garage, it seems as though I have come full circle. The great difference is that my health and the health of my family doesn't depend on endless numbers of opinions and scientific studies. Our health depends on Him as we walk in the steps which He has ordered.

> Bless our God, O peoples, And sound His praise abroad, Who keeps us in life, And does not allow our feet to slip. (Ps. 66:8)

At this juncture, it is important to emphasize that this is not a book about the forbidding of meat. It is a book about submitting our will to God in our choice of foods. We cannot even evaluate the choices which are available unless we are willing to walk in wisdom, according to the leading of the Spirit, and not according to the desires of the flesh. The Word of God is clear on the matter of forbidding meat:

> But the Spirit explicitly says that in later times some will fall away from the faith, paying attention to deceitful spirits and doctrines of demons,
>
> by means of the hypocrisy of liars seared in their own conscience as with a branding iron,
>
> men who forbid marriage and advocate abstaining from foods, which God has created to be gratefully shared in by those who believe and know the truth.
>
> For everything created by God is good, and nothing is to be rejected if it is received with gratitude:
>
> for it is sanctified by means of the word of God and prayer. (1 Tim. 4:1-5)

We know that meat was not in God's original diet for man. He only included meat after the flood:

> And the fear of you and the terror of you shall be on every beast of the earth and on every bird of the sky: with everything that creeps on the ground, and all the fish of the sea, into your hand they are given.
>
> Every moving thing that is alive shall be food for you; I give all to you, as I gave the green plant.
>
> Only you shall not eat flesh with its life, that is its blood. (Gen. 9:2-4)

It is important to remember that the Lord also allows His children—in both the Old Testament and the New Testament—to refrain from eating meat. Clearly, we are free to choose a vegetarian diet. It is important to note some specific examples. The first diet recorded in Genesis only included food from the plant kingdom. Then God said, "Behold, I have given you every plant yielding seed that is on the surface of all the earth, and every tree which has fruit yielding seed; it shall be food for you" (Gen. 1:29).

Daniel is a notable example. He asked that the overseer let him and his three friends eat vegetables and drink water.

> Then let our appearance be observed in your presence, and the appearance of the youths who are eating the king's choice food; and deal with your servants according to what you see. (Dan. 1:13)
>
> And at the end of ten days their appearance seemed better and they were fatter than all the youths who had been eating the king's choice food. (Dan. 1:15)
>
> And as for these four youths, God gave them knowledge and intelligence in every branch of literature and wisdom; Daniel even understood all kinds of visions and dreams. (Dan. 1:17)
>
> And the king talked with them, and out of them all not one was found like Daniel, Hananiah, Mishael

and Azariah; so they entered the king's personal
service. (Dan. 1:19)

The Apostle Paul makes it clear that we are not to
judge one another concerning what we decide is best to
eat. I have heard preachers state that it is unscriptural to
abstain from meat. The Word clearly says we may eat
according to our faith:

> One man has faith that he may eat all things, but
> he who is weak eats vegetables only.

> Let not him who eats regard with contempt him
> who does not eat, and let not him who does not
> eat judge him who eats, for God has accepted
> him. (Rom. 14:2–3)

When I think of the words "he who is weak eats vegetables only," I am reminded that it does not say, "he who
is weak in faith eats vegetables only." Though we are weak
in the flesh, we become strong by the power of God. Anyone whose health and strength are declining is weak. I
believe that until that person is strong again, it is best to
avoid eating meat. Many of us who are enjoying strength
and vitality on an entirely vegetarian regime do not want
to eat meat, poultry, or fish again.

As Christians, we are free to eat meat or not to eat
meat. But, as Dr. Mary Ruth Swope says, "We are not free
to choose the consequences that will result."[15] And, in later
chapters, we will learn that consequences do result from
the choices which we make.

Also, in later chapters, we will discuss foods which
build health and products which destroy our health. In
Part One, I have disclosed my personal choices. I believe
that it is important to relate the way in which God delivers
us even as we walk in ignorance. When I consider the
amount of canned red salmon that I ate during a two-year
period, I shudder. According to Dr. Neal Barnard, indus-
trial chemicals called PCBs have been found in 43 percent
of the salmon; PCBs are linked with cancer and are particularly threatening for a developing fetus.[16] Dr. Barnard

cites *Consumer Reports* as the primary resource on the quantity of PCBs in salmon. He recommends that women stop eating fish years before they become pregnant, because PCB and mercury contamination are so common in fish. PCBs can remain in the body for decades.[17]

In Part Two, I discuss the choices that numbers of other people have made. Now, in the nineties, people who were suffering and dying from degenerative diseases are alive and active. We need to understand how we can walk in health simply by changing the way that we eat and the way that we think. And, everyone needs to understand the way in which grains, legumes, vegetables, and fruits build healthy cells in our bodies and enable our bodies to fight disease. The research which supports my present choices appears in the following chapters. Our environment has been polluted. We need to evaluate the quality of our air, water, and food and find ways in which we can protect ourselves and ways in which we can compensate for the damage done to the world in which we must live. At the very least, we must ask ourselves if the foods we are eating and drinking are the wholesome foods which God intended. If they are not, He will deliver us from our desire for them. He is the source of strength and peace. The Lord will give strength to His people; The Lord will bless His people with peace (Ps. 29:11).

Part Two

Biblical Steps to Optimal Health and Nutrition

He sent His word and healed them and delivered them from their destructions.

Let them give thanks to the Lord for His lovingkindness,

And for His wonders to the sons of men!

Let them also offer sacrifices of thanksgiving,

And tell of his works with joyful singing.

—Psalms 107:20–22

Become a Thankful and Joyful Person

Preparation:

Embrace your circumstances

Confess and repent

Offer a sacrifice of thanksgiving

Sing praise and shout for joy

Be renewed in the spirit of your mind

Embrace Your Circumstances

Scientific research clearly reveals that our thoughts and feelings alter our biochemistry. As Christians, we know that is true simply because the Word of God declares that it is true.

A joyful heart is good medicine,
But a broken spirit dries up the bones. (Ps. 17:22)

A soothing tongue is a tree of life, But perversion in it crushes the spirit. (Prov. 15:4)

The tongue of the wise brings healing. (Prov. 12:18)

Dr. S. I. McMillen, college physician, medical missionary, and writer of the Christian classic, *None of These Diseases*, presents an important case for devoting our energies to the Kingdom of God, rather than seeking great things for ourselves. The book is not about how to eat; it is about how to think. He sites a 1955 report from *Health News* in which the New York State Department of Health published photographs of two human adrenal glands. One gland was

normal in size, while the other gland had hypertrophied.
The latter was greatly enlarged. Dr. McMillen makes these
observations:

> The individual from whom the enlarged gland was
> removed probably died many years ahead of his
> time because the increased supply of adrenaline
> played havoc with one or more of his bodily func-
> tions. He not only shortened his days, but his days
> were likely filled with emotional turmoil. . . . If a
> person sits at high noon in the security of his own
> home and allows his mind to think of burglars and
> charging bulls, his emotional center will send out
> identical alarm messages to the glands, heart and
> blood-pressure centers, as it would if the individual
> were actually attacked. Although the body needs an
> excess of hormones for genuine emergency situa-
> tions, an excessive and frequent production of hor-
> mones over weeks and months results in deleteri-
> ous responses.[1]

Dr. McMillen teaches simply that poor health is usually
the result of our carnal nature, and that health and genu-
ine happiness result when our thoughts and attitudes conform with the teachings of the Bible.

Today—as scientific studies verify McMillen's conclusions regarding the effect of the mind on the body—physicians, scientists, and educators offer many different "stress
management" techniques. Many Christians in the medical
profession now offer the wisdom of the Bible in counseling patients to change their thought lives. Many Christian
physicians work with biblical counselors. It is heartening to
know that their patients are able first, to find redemption
in Christ and, second, healing through the power and
principles of His Word.

Other health professionals offer the Bible as one of
many contrasting approaches to peace and happiness. For
them, all paths lead to God. Educational resources abound
which tell us how to relax, how to breathe, how to develop
inner peace, and how to cultivate interpersonal relationships. And, while many of these books have interesting and

useful ideas, we need first to focus on the Book that is essential.

My husband and I are particularly interested in hearing from those in the medical profession who recognize that the study of nutrition is vital to the practice of medicine. We are grateful that there exists a Physicians Committee for Responsible Medicine, and we appreciate the important work that these health professionals are doing. But, as we recommend their books and studies, we acknowledge that many members of that organization may not share our faith in the Lord Jesus Christ. Therefore, in reading the books written by those men and women, we need to pay close attention to their comments regarding human behavior. No counselor can offer life-giving advice unless he knows the Counselor who is the Giver of Life. Physicians who suggest that there are many ways to God and that all religions are valid are not the physicians to approach for counsel regarding our thoughts and behaviors. Christ Himself refutes all such teaching:

> I am the way, and the truth, and the life; no one comes to the Father, but through Me. If you had known Me, you would have known my Father also; from now on you have known Him, and have seen Him. (John 14:6–7)

We are very grateful for Dr. Dean Ornish's book, *Dr. Dean Ornish's Program for Reversing Heart Disease; The Only System Scientifically Proven to Reverse Heart Disease Without Drugs or Surgery.*[2] We believe that his book will encourage many people to make choices which will save their lives. Although we don't share the philosophical and religious views which he expresses in the chapters concerning behavioral management, we recommend this book most highly.

The Scripture presents a startlingly different view of what we call "stress" and our certainty that we must "manage" it. If we look closely at the Word of God, we see that the whole notion of "stress management" may be something of a distraction. What is it we call "stressful"? We are only talking about circumstances. The baby is screaming; the house burns down; the toilet overflows; our spouse dies; the neighbors are unfriendly; the paycheck stops; a child goes blind. Do we really imagine that the circumstances of life call for "stress management techniques"? In all of life's challenges—great and small—we need Him. We need His divine nature. He promises to change our carnal nature if we come to Him in faith and repentance. He promises to purify our hearts.

As children of God, we know that every circumstance in our lives has a purpose and a plan. He uses all of the happy and unhappy events of our lives to conform us to His image (Rom. 8:29). I did not know the truth of Romans 8:29 until my first husband died. My prayers were arguments with God. I could not, I would not, accept the circumstances. The finality of death tormented me. I could do nothing, absolutely nothing to alter the finality of death. But, I submitted to His Word. And, one day in May of 1978, not quite two months after Frank died, I read Romans chapter 8 as though for the first time. I saw the truth; I believed it; I realized that God loved Frank and God loved me! I would come to love His plan.

Deep breathing exercises and relaxation techniques are temporary measures. We need to go to God for the deep work. Those times when we find ourselves upset by minor annoyances, or nervous and undone in the face of great difficulties, the problem is our carnal nature. Stress management techniques will help us feel better, work better, accomplish more. But, we must be sure that we incorporate those techniques into the real business of our lives—allowing His Word to come alive in our hearts. The importance of "stressful circumstances" is that they allow us to discover who we are. Only through the circumstances of life do we recognize our sinful nature. Recognizing our failure is liberating! It is only through fear and unbelief that we deny our sin. When we repent and confess, we find ourselves safely in His arms.

Let's look at a sublime example of how to respond to hardship. When the greatest trials come, who we are in Christ transforms us through the very agony of the event. Imagine Stephen as his persecutors became enraged by him. The Word says that "being full of the Holy Spirit, he gazed intently into heaven and saw the glory of God, and Jesus standing at the right hand of God" (Acts 7:55). What God gave to Stephen in a vision, He gives to us in His Word. And, by the power of the Holy Spirit, we can see the glory of God and Jesus standing at the right hand of God! Remember when Jesus said to Martha, "Did I not say to you, if you believe, you will see the glory of God?" (John 11:40). If we believe, we will see the glory of God.

The same grace He gave Stephen is freely available to us. How foolish we are when we fail to ask and receive. As they stoned Stephen, they laid their robes aside at the feet of a young man named Saul "who was in hearty agreement with putting him to death" (Acts 8:1). How thrilling to consider that "Saul, still breathing threats and murder against the Lord" was soon to meet the Lord!

> Suddenly a light from heaven flashed around him; and he fell to the ground, and heard a voice saying to him, "Saul, Saul. why are you persecuting Me?" And He said, "Who art Thou, Lord?" And he said, "I am Jesus whom you are persecuting, but rise, and enter the city, and it shall be told you what you must do." (Acts 9:6)

How wonderful for us that God chose Saul, a murderer of Christians, and changed him into the Apostle Paul. Through his writings, inspired by the Holy Spirit, we can understand faith and grace. God gave us Paul as an example of complete victory in Him. Faith is that victory. The life of the Apostle Paul gives real significance to the word *stress* as we use it. When we see difficulties through his eyes, we see only the Kingdom of God. He didn't endure hardship, he embraced it. Paul was not delivered from his thorn in the flesh. And yet, he found his circumstances reasonable, acceptable, and a cause for gladness.

For the Lord said to him, "My grace is sufficient for you, for power is perfected in weakness." To the Lord's words he responds:

> Most gladly, therefore, I will rather boast about my weaknesses, that the power of Christ may dwell in me. Therefore I am well content with weaknesses, with insults, with distresses, with persecutions, with difficulties, for Christ's sake; for when I am weak, then I am strong. (2 Cor. 12:9-10)

Even Christian writers tell us to "manage stress" by making sure that we have proper rest and diversions. They suggest making time for recreation, such as hobbies and sports activities. But, that advice only works for those who have the financial freedom to deliver themselves from all that is stressful. What about men, women, and children in other cultures whose idea of a good day is being able to find enough food to stay alive. And, what about the families in this country who have to work hard just to make enough money for the essentials. Praise God that although we may have little or no money for diversions, we may have His peace. God's Word is for the rich and the poor. His answers don't depend on circumventing circumstances. He walked Paul through great difficulties that our hearts might rise with the knowledge that He will enable us to meet every situation by His grace.

> I have learned to be content in whatever circumstances I am. I know how to get along with humble means, and I also know how to live in prosperity; in any and every circumstance I have learned the secret of being filled and going hungry, both of having abundance and suffering need. I can do all things through Him who strengthens me. (Phil. 4:11-13)

Life could not shake or shatter Paul, because Paul was secure in Him. To those of us walking in need he says, "And my God shall supply all your needs according to His riches in glory in Christ Jesus" (Phil. 4:19).

Confess and Repent

Confessing, repenting, and receiving His grace and mercy are the basis of every victory in Christ which we enjoy. The Word cleanses us as the Holy Spirit prepares our hearts. The Lord Himself tells us in John 15:3 that we are clean because of the Word that He has spoken to us. The faith which brings forth our redemption comes into our hearts by the power of His Word. "So faith comes through hearing, and hearing by the word of Christ" (Rom. 10:17).

> For you have been born again not of seed which is perishable but imperishable, that is, through the living and abiding word of God. (1 Pet. 1:23)

Then, as Christians, the Word enables us to become like Him: "Christ also loved the church and gave Himself up for her; that He might present to Himself the church in all her glory, having no spot or wrinkle or any such thing; but that she should be holy and blameless" (Eph. 5:25–27).

We know that changing our hearts and minds is not only possible through Christ, His Word commands that we change. The Apostle Paul tells us why we may have this hope:

> For this reason, I bow my knees before the Father, from whom every family in heaven and earth derives its name, that He would grant you, according to the riches of His glory, to be strengthened with Power through His spirit in the inner man; so that Christ may dwell in your hearts through faith; and that you, being rooted and grounded in love, may be able to comprehend with all the saints what is the breadth and length and height and depth, and to know the love of Christ which surpasses knowledge, that you may be filled up to all the fullness of God. (Eph. 3:14–19)

Only through the power of His Word can we turn our fear to faith. Although we may know that the excessive production of hormones causes arthritis, mental illness, vascular disease, gastrointestinal disease, fatigue, injury, and tension, we cannot make ourselves unfearful. We need Him. And, what about our selfishness and our self-centeredness? Only by His love can we become a giver and not a taker. We become givers by bowing our knees before the Father. He enables us to partake in the riches of His glory. Our lives are only transformed by confession, repentance, and prayer. And, we may come before His throne boldly, in the name of our Lord and Savior, again and again.

> Let us therefore draw near with confidence to the throne of grace, that we may receive mercy and may find grace to help in time of need. (Heb. 4:16)

We are delivered from evil, cleansed from all unrighteousness, by the blood of Christ. Thus, the Word of God prepares our hearts and enables us to be thankful.

Offer a Sacrifice of Thanksgiving

Because God tells us to offer a sacrifice of thanksgiving, we must obey if we are to walk in His blessings. We also need to be honest and realize that many of us are unthankful quite often. And, as Christians, it is very easy to walk in denial. We say to ourselves, "That is wrong. I won't do it," when in fact we have already done it. We may awaken with ungrateful hearts and say, "I know it is a sin to be unthankful. I do not want to sin; therefore, I won't be unthankful." If we ask the Lord to reveal our hearts to us, He will. He already knows our hearts! Then, our conversations with ourselves and with Him are different. "Lord, I feel a heaviness. Somehow my joy and gladness are gone. As I read your Word, please change my heart. Give me your thoughts. Out of my will, I praise You and I thank You." Liberation from sin comes with confession. After we confess our sin, we must trust in the Lord, and in Him alone, to deliver us from the bondage of sin by the power of His Word. For many of us, a rainy day can make us unthankful, the slightest inconvenience can make us unthankful. And yet, He loves us. If we open our hearts to Him, He will change us.

> Just as a father has compassion on his children, So the Lord has compassion on those who fear Him. For He Himself knows our frame, He is mindful that we are but dust. (Ps. 103:13–14)

God tells us specifically to offer a "sacrifice of thanksgiving." If we were already "feeling thankful," then He would not tell us to offer a "sacrifice." He understands our weaknesses and failures. Life is filled with disappointments, tragedy, and inconveniences. But, we can learn to embrace those trials if we are walking in Him. That is the benefit, the result of justification. These wonderful verses are familiar to many of us, but are they alive in us? If they are alive in us then they never grow old.

> We have obtained our introduction by faith into this grace in which we stand; and we exult in hope of the glory of God. And not only this, but we also exult in our tribulations, knowing that tribulation brings about perseverance; and perseverance, proven character; and proven character, hope; and hope does not disappoint, because the love of God has been poured out within our hearts through the Holy Spirit who was given us. (Rom. 5:2–5)

Seeking distractions from our "stress" is very different from exulting in our tribulations. The goal of the rest, relaxation, and diversion strategies is comfort. But, tribulation has another purpose—building character. The tennis court, the evening out, the vacation may be useful in our lives. But, they aren't useful as a means of enabling us to bear our problems. Again, what about those who cannot afford to divert themselves with pleasantries. Is God unfair? No! He will enable us to exult in our tribulation. The circumstances have meaning. They are part of His plan. If we trust the Planner, we can trust the plan.

Offer to God a sacrifice of thanksgiving, And pay
your vows to the Most High;

And call upon Me in the day of trouble;
I shall rescue you, and you will honor Me. (Ps. 50:14–
15)

Then by faith, we speak His Word and obey: "To Thee
I shall offer a sacrifice of thanksgiving, and call upon the
name of the Lord" (Ps. 116:17).

Sing Praise and Shout for Joy

If we are willing to be cleansed by the Word and offer
a sacrifice of thanksgiving, then we will obey His command
that we sing praise and shout for joy. All men are exhorted
to praise God. And, the psalm which many of us know
from childhood, Psalm 100, tells us how to enter His gates
and His courts.

Shout joyfully to the Lord, all the earth.
Serve the Lord with gladness;
Come before Him with joyful singing.
Know that the Lord Himself is God;
It is He who has made us and not we ourselves;
We are His people and the sheep of His pasture.

Enter His gates with thanksgiving,
And His courts with praise.
Give thanks to Him; bless His name.
For the Lord is good;
His lovingkindness is everlasting,
And His faithfulness to all generations. (Ps. 100)

The one emotion that seems to have the greatest negative impact on our immune system is loneliness. We all
benefit from having a "healthy mental attitude," but the
only certain way to have thoughts that heal is to think His
thoughts. According to Psalm 100, we need never be lonely.
We are His sheep, loved with an everlasting love. And He
tells us how to come close to Him, how to enter His gates
and enter His courts. But, we must remind ourselves of the
truth. The psalmist gives specific reasons for singing His
praises:

He hath dealt bountifully with me. (Ps. 13:6, KJV) Thou hast turned for me my mourning into dancing; Thou hast put off my sackcloth, and girded me with gladness. (Ps. 30:11, KJV)

I will sing of Thy power; yea, I will sing aloud of Thy mercy in the morning: for Thou hast been my defense and refuge in the day of trouble. Unto thee, O my strength, will I sing: for God is my defense, and the God of my mercy. (Ps. 59:16, KJV)

So will I sing praise unto Thy name for ever, that I may daily perform my vows. (Ps. 61:8, KJV)

It is a good thing to give thanks unto the Lord, and to sing praises unto Thy name, O Most High: to show forth Thy lovingkindness in the morning, and thy faithfulness every night. (Ps. 92:1-2, KJV)

O come, let us sing unto the Lord; let us make a joyful noise to the rock of our salvation. Let us come before his presence with thanksgiving, and make a joyful noise to the rock of our salvation. (Ps. 95:1, KJV)

Sing unto him, sing psalms unto him: talk ye of all his wondrous works. (Ps. 105:2, KJV)

I will sing praises unto my God while I have any being. (Ps. 146:2, KJV)

The psalmist tells us that hope is in His Word, that the entrance of His Word gives light, that it gives understanding to the simple (Ps. 119: 130). Singing that truth strengthens our bodies. There are peptides throughout our bodies. They are present in the white blood cells which make up our immune system. Our emotions literally produce natural peptides which strengthen our immune system. As we have mentioned, our emotions also produce hormones which change our body chemistry. Some hormones facilitate healing, while others promote disease.[3] God's Word ought to excite us. That is why He tells us to rejoice in Him and to shout with joy. The benefit of that excitement is that rejoicing has a biochemical effect on our bodies, sending hormones that promote health and healing. Rejoicing strengthens and heals our bodies at the cellular level.

> Be glad in the Lord and rejoice you righteous ones.
> And shout for joy all you who are upright in heart.
> (Ps. 32:11)

> Rejoice always; pray without ceasing; in everything give thanks; for this is God's will for you in Christ Jesus. (1 Thess. 5:16–18)

In the morning, listening to Scripture in song, the children and I move about the room singing with the words and music. We use the large muscle groups. We swing our arms and lift our feet continuously and rhythmically. We are able to learn the Scriptures readily because we are singing them. Our thoughts are elevated, and our feelings are aroused by His Word. The music lifts our hearts. And, we ought not be ashamed to say our feelings are "aroused." How can we read or speak or sing, "Bless the Lord, O my soul; And all that is within me, bless His holy name" (Ps. 103:1) and not be moved!

I have talked to many, many people who find it a struggle to establish a regular quiet time every morning. Perhaps part of the problem is that it starts out "quiet." When we sing hymns and spiritual songs and praise Him in joyful song, something happens in our hearts. We awaken—body, mind, and spirit—to the Kingdom of God. It is essential, no matter how old or young we are, to hear the Word of God sung and spoken with passion and zeal. Our dear friend, Dr. Al Smith, founder of Singspiration, has dedicated his life to publishing, composing, and arranging gospel songs and choruses. He inspires congregations to begin singing together again, with joy and gladness. And he urges people to keep their hearts encouraged throughout the week by playing and singing gospel choruses in their homes. He has written so many songs we sing, but his sweet chorus based on Psalm 113:3 is a wonderful way to begin and end the day:

His name shall be praised, His name shall be praised
His name shall be praised hallelujah! From the ris-
ing of the sun, until the day is done His Name, His
Name shall be praised![4]

When we begin singing in our homes, it is often easier
with small children. They give us an excuse to make it an
event. But, all of us need to sing praise and shout for joy
as we worship Him alone each day. Then, as the words and
melodies become fixed in our minds, iniquity loses dominion over us. His precepts deliver us from oppressive people;
His precepts revive us, body and soul.

> Establish my footsteps in Thy word, And do not let
> any iniquity have dominion over me. Redeem me
> from the oppression of man, That I may keep Thy
> precepts. (Ps. 119:133–134)

> I will never forget Thy precepts, For by them Thou
> hast revived me. (Ps. 119:93)

Toxins are released from our bodies as we exercise,
and we are filled with energy. But, our main purpose is not
to exercise; it is to praise and glorify the Lord! Whether we
are old or young, alone or with our families, we can enjoy
this time of worship in the privacy of our homes. We are
unhindered and undistracted. And, just as the Lord ad-
monishes us to offer Him a sacrifice of thanksgiving and
to come before Him singing and shouting; He exhorts us
to move about, to dance before Him.

> Let them praise His name with dancing. (Ps. 149:3)

> Praise Him with timbrel and dancing. (Ps. 150:4)

Some may be in wheelchairs and can only swing their
arms. Some may not be able to move any muscles at all.
Many can walk and sing and shout. Others can dance. But,
all of us can make melody in our hearts and bless the Lord
with all that is within us, for He is worthy of our praise.

Be Renewed in the Spirit of Your Mind

By faith we are empowered by the Holy Spirit to do God's will. But, it is the flesh of man that seeks to manipulate circumstances through the power of positive thinking. There are many resources available which explore ways to cultivate a positive mental attitude. Now that research clearly indicates that our attitudes impact our biochemistry, more people want to know how to think "healthy thoughts." Scientific studies indicate that "positive" thoughts make people more productive and energetic, and "negative thoughts lead to failure and dissatisfaction." In popular magazines, a positive mental attitude is associated with physical and mental health, as well as financial success. Articles portray "well-rounded" and "successful" people as ones who are physically fit, committed to some form of regular exercise, involved in meaningful relationships, and able to manage their time. Successful people are often characterized as well-rested and financially able to enjoy the hobbies, sports, and diversions which they most enjoy.

Some Christian writers speak of the "power of positive thinking" as though it were a biblical way to improve our lives. Certainly, our thoughts shape our lives. "For as he thinks within himself, so is he" (Prov. 23:7). And, surely our fears have the creative power to bring down all that faith seeks to uphold. Job's lament is that "what I fear comes upon me, And what I dread befalls me" (Job 3:25). But, in what or whom do we place our trust—God or our positive thoughts? And, whose will do we seek to accomplish? Are we trusting the power of our positive thoughts to accomplish our will? If we are empowered by the Holy Spirit, then we walk in the will of God and glorify His name. Romans 8:28 is a "positive promise" to Christians that "God causes all things to work together for good to those who love God, to those who are called according to His purpose. For whom He foreknew, He also predestined to become conformed to the image of His Son." Galatians 5:22–24 tells us that the fruit of the Spirit produces "positive" character qualities which enable the Christian to walk in newness of life every day:

> The fruit of the Spirit is love, joy, peace, patience, kindness, goodness, faithfulness, gentleness, self-control; against such things there is no law. Now those who belong to Christ Jesus have crucified the flesh with its passions and desires.

Recently, I attended a delightful conference sponsored by a Christian organization. In one of the meetings, a group of people ended their presentation with a creed, a list of positive imperatives. The people reading this list were kind, gentle people whom I believe seek to live in accordance with these values. But, after their presentation, a heaviness fell over me, and I began to consider the admonitions in the creed that they read. We cannot walk in accordance with such a creed without the power of God. Everything we are and everything we do depends upon the mercy of God.

> For He says to Moses, "I will have mercy on whom I have mercy, and I will have compassion on whom I have compassion." So then it does not depend on the man who wills or the man who runs, but on God who has mercy. (Rom. 9:15–16)

Unless we seek His power and mercy we will not be able to walk in His eternal way. Without Him, nothing that we are and nothing that we do has light or life:

> For the mind set on the flesh is death, but the mind set on the Spirit is life and peace, because the mind set on the flesh is hostile toward God; for it does not subject itself to the law of God, for it is not even able to do so, and those who are in the flesh cannot please God. However, you are not in the flesh but in the Spirit if indeed the Spirit of God dwells in you. But if anyone does not have the Spirit of Christ, he does not belong to Him. (Rom. 8:6–9)

When I came home, I wrote a summary of the creed. The words indicate that man can determine his own destiny. By exalting man, rather than bowing before the Father, we blaspheme His holy name. The creed is deceptively upbeat and right sounding:

> Look at the bright side of everything and make your good thoughts come into being; be strong and peaceful—never worried, never angry, never fearful; speak of health, happiness, and prosperity; be cheerful around other people and be enthusiastic about the events of their lives; forget about your own failures and work on greater accomplishments; never criticize others, instead think of the good in them; acknowledge God as the source of everything in your life.

But, those imperatives leave out the plea for mercy, pardon, and deliverance. We haven't the power to walk out such commands in the flesh! We either fall into despair or self-deception. Many are honest enough not to attempt such perfection without Almighty God. If we truly acknowledge God as the source of everything, then we will seek His wisdom and power in all that we do. Then, by His strength and grace, goodness and mercy shall follow us all the days of our lives, and we will dwell in the house of the Lord forever (Ps. 23:6).

The power to do good does not come through positive thoughts, it comes through the blood of the Lord Jesus. When we receive His death on the cross as the payment for our sin, we come into a personal relationship with Jesus our Savior. We become a child of God the Father, comforted by the Holy Spirit. "For in Him all the fullness of deity dwells in bodily form" (Col. 2:9). God has a remedy for our sin, for our inability to understand what is good and to accomplish it.

> He made Him who knew no sin to be sin on our behalf, that we might become the righteousness of God in Him. (2 Cor. 5:21)

We begin by confessing with our mouths Jesus as Lord and believing with our hearts that God raised Him from the dead.

For with the heart man believes, resulting in righteousness, and with the mouth he confesses resulting in salvation. (Rom. 10:10)

With God's promises come peace, because we are saved and delivered from all unrighteousness by His grace. We can embrace the challenges of His Word because He is careful to perform His Word (Jer. 1:12).

By Obeying God's Commands, We Can Rest in His Promises

His Peace:

Rejoice in the Lord always; again I say rejoice.

Let your forbearing spirit be known to all men, The Lord is near.

Be anxious for nothing, but by prayer and supplication with thanksgiving let your requests be made known to God.

And the peace of God, which surpasses all comprehension, shall guard your hearts and your minds in Christ Jesus.

Whatever is true, whatever is honorable, whatever is right, whatever is pure, whatever is lovely, whatever is of good repute, if there is any excellence and if anything worthy of praise, let your mind dwell on these things.

. . . Practice these things; and the God of peace shall be with you. (Phil. 4:4–9)

His Healing:

Give attention to my words; Incline your ear to my sayings. Do not let them depart from your sight; Keep them in the midst of your heart.

For they are life to those who find them, And health to all their whole body. (Prov. 4:20–22)

The tongue of the wise brings healing. (Prov. 12:18)

His Friendship:

A friend loves at all times. (Prov. 17:7)

Do you not know that friendship with the world is hostility toward God? Therefore whoever wishes to be a friend of the world makes himself an enemy of God. (James 4:4)

Greater love has no one than this, that one lay down his life for his friends. You are my friends, if you do what I command you. No longer do I call you slaves, for the slave does not know what his master is doing; but I have called you friends, for all things that I have heard from My Father I have made known to you.

You did not choose Me, but I chose you, and appointed you, that you should bear fruit, and that your fruit should remain, that whatever you ask of the Father in My name, He may give to you.

This I command you, that you love one another. (John 15:13–17)

Do not associate with a man given to anger; Or go with a hot-tempered man, Lest you learn his ways, And find a snare for yourself. (Prov. 22:24–25)

Do not be deceived: "Bad company corrupts good morals." (1 Cor. 15:33)

Faith, Gift of God:

Now faith is the assurance of things hoped for, the conviction of things unseen. (Heb. 11:1)

Our Purpose in Him:

Brethren, I do not regard myself as having laid hold of it yet; but one thing I do: forgetting what lies behind and reaching forward to what lies ahead.

I press on toward the goal for the prize of the upward call of God in Christ Jesus. (Phil. 3:13–14)

Our Conduct in Christ:

> And we urge you brethren, admonish the unruly, encourage the fainthearted, help the weak, be patient with all men. See to it that no one repays evil for evil, but always seek after that which is good for one another and for all men. (1 Thess. 5:23–24)

> Love is patient, love is kind, and is not jealous; love does not brag and is not arrogant, does not act unbecomingly; it does not seek its own, is not provoked, does not take into account a wrong suffered, does not rejoice in unrighteousness, but rejoices in the truth; bears all things, believes all things, hopes all things, endures all things. (1 Cor. 13:4–7)

> Now may the God of peace Himself sanctify you entirely; and may your spirit and soul and body be preserved complete, without blame at the coming of our Lord Jesus Christ.

> Faithful is He who calls you, and He also will bring it to pass. (1 Thess. 5:23–24)

> Love never fails. (1 Cor. 13:8)

When we are empowered by the Holy Spirit, we have the mind of Christ concerning peace, healing and health, friendship, faith, purpose, and conduct. In Him we do not seek to control our lives and determine events. By His Spirit, we walk in obedience to God's Word.

We can become thankful and joyful people, people who can embrace the circumstances of our lives and exult in tribulation. The next four steps to optimal health and nutrition will be an absolute joy for those who receive the teaching of this first step. And, the teaching is His. He does the changing; we have only to cry out and ask to be changed.

> Let us run with endurance the race that is set before us, fixing our eyes on Jesus, the author and perfecter of faith, who for the joy set before Him endured the cross, despising the shame, and has sat down at the right hand of the throne of God. (Heb. 12:1–2)

Enjoy Preparing, Serving, and Eating Foods Which Are Essential for Optimal Health

Preparation:

Recognize the ways in which the 1956 USDA Dietary Guidelines have impacted our culture and influenced the food choices of two generations of Americans.

Consider the scientific research carefully to determine whether you should eat meat, poultry, fish, eggs, and dairy in moderation or whether you should avoid those foods completely.

Appreciate the delicious array of foods which God has provided for optimal health and nutrition.

Learn to identify "deceptive foods" and purpose not to consume them.

Locate reliable whole foods suppliers.

Stock the pantry with foods for life.

Learn to prepare and present life-giving foods which appeal to both the eye and the palate.

Dietary Guidelines Followed by the General Population Since World War II

Before we discuss the wide range of delicious, health-building foods which are available, we need to explore three topics: 1) the specific dietary guidelines which the United States Department of Agriculture has issued, 2) the way in which those guidelines have impacted the health science curricula in the United States, and 3) the scientific studies which have prompted leaders in the fields of nutrition, science, and medicine to abandon the United States Department of Agriculture's Dietary Guidelines and to issue guidelines of their own. Before we reject the information which we learned during health science class in school, most of us want to evaluate the credibility of the new information. We also need to examine the extent to which the encyclopedias and textbooks in the fifties, sixties, seventies, and eighties relied on the USDA Dietary Guidelines as a credible source of vital information on health and nutrition. An entire generation of Americans learned how to eat based on the United States Department of Agriculture's Dietary Guidelines, and that generation taught another generation to do the same. Dr. Neal Barnard, president of the Physicians Committee for Responsible Medicine and member of the faculty of George Washington University School of Medicine, comments on the consequences of the poor training in health and nutrition which Americans have received:

> The results are tragic. There are 4,000 heart attacks every single day in this country. The traditional four food groups and the eating patterns they prescribed have led to cancer and heart disease in epidemic numbers, and have killed more people than any other factor in America. More then automobile accidents, more than tobacco, more than all the wars of this century combined.[1]

In 1916, the USDA introduced the first food guide, *Food for Young Children*. By 1946, public health workers and public school teachers taught and promoted the Basic Seven Food Groups, which were presented in a wheel. Most of us who are over forty years old have been influenced somewhat by the Basic Seven Food Groups because that is the nutritional system our parents learned. And, although we now know that these guidelines are not the basis for optimal health, they are safer by far than the United States Department of Agriculture's Four Food Groups which replaced the Basic Seven. In the Basic Seven system, four of the groups cover fruits, vegetables, and grains. Also, a distinction is made between raw and cooked vegetables.

> Group One—Meats, poultry, fish, eggs, dried beans and peas, and nuts
>
> Group Two—Leafy green and yellow vegetables
>
> Group Three—Citrus fruits, raw cabbage, salad greens, and tomatoes
>
> Group Four—Potatoes and other vegetables, and non-citrus fruits
>
> Group Five—Breads, cereals, and flour
>
> Group Six—Butter and fortified margarines
>
> Group Seven—Milk and milk products

Nutritionists advocating the Basic Seven system suggested that a child should have three or more glasses of milk each day and that a teen-ager should have four or more glasses. They recommended one daily serving from each of the remaining six groups.[2] We will examine the subject of milk consumption later in this chapter. Many nutritionists continued using the Basic Seven Food Groups long after the USDA changed their guidelines.

In 1956, the United States Department of Agriculture introduced the Four Food Groups. The amount of fat and cholesterol in meals drastically increased as a result of this system:

> Group One—The milk group
>
> Group Two—The meat group
>
> Group Three—The fruit and vegetable group
>
> Group Four—The bread and cereal group

The *World Book Encyclopedia*, 1966 edition, features a complete teaching of the Basic Seven Food Groups and offers a relatively short explanation of the Four Food Groups which had been introduced by the U. S. Department of Agriculture in 1956.[3] That indicates that in the opinions of the editors, the value of the older Basic Seven

Food Groups system could not be ignored. Clearly, some nutritionists did not consider the Basic Four an improvement over the earlier guidelines. The 1966, *World Book* refers to the Four Food Groups as "A Daily Food Plan":

> A Daily Food Plan can be used in place of the Basic Seven. Nutritionists suggest four or more servings daily from the vegetable-fruit and bread-cereal groups, and two servings from the meat group. Children should drink three or more cups of milk a day, and adults two or more. Butter, margarine, sugar, oils, and other foods not in the plan are also important to health.[4]

Textbook publishers such as Laidlaw Brothers in their 1980 edition of *Keeping Healthy*[5] and Scott, Foresman and Company in their 1971 edition of *Health and Growth 2*[6] are typical of the publishers of health science curricula for the public schools. They offer the United States Department of Agriculture's Guidelines exclusively as the best information available regarding health and nutrition. The Scott, Foresman text, featuring photographs of each food group provided by the National Dairy Council, shows cheese, milk, ice cream, and cottage cheese in the first group; ham, beef (various cuts of red meat), chicken, eggs, beans, and nuts in the second; fruits and vegetables in the third; and bread, crackers, cereals, and pasta in the fourth.[7] Here's a daily menu suggested by the Laidlaw text.[8]

Breakfast: Fruit or fruit juice
Bread or cereal
Eggs or meat (lean bacon or ham)

Lunch: Meat or sandwiches (with meat or peanut butter)
Vegetables or soup
Fruit or fruit juices
Milk

Dinner: Meat
Vegetables (cooked or in a salad)
Bread
Milk

Just after the Physicians Committee for Responsible Medicine released the information about their New Four Food Groups in 1991, the United States Department of Agriculture released the details about its own new plan. The outraged meat and dairy industries forced the Department of Agriculture to reconsider the graphic, which delayed the release of the food guide for nearly a year.[9]

The 1992 USDA Food Guide Pyramid that eventually made its appearance because the United States Department of Agriculture could no longer deny the findings of numerous research studies linking diet and disease: some dietary regimes cause degenerative disease, while other health strategies actually prevent, or even cure, many illnesses. The 1992 USDA Food Guide Pyramid de-emphasizes animal products in favor of whole grains, fruits, and vegetables. At the base of the pyramid is the bread, cereal, rice, and pasta group, with a recommendation of six to eleven servings. At the second level are the fruit group (with two servings) and the vegetable group (with three to five servings); on the third level are the milk, yogurt, and cheese group (with two to three servings) and the meat, poultry, fish, dry beans, eggs, and nuts group (with two to four servings). At the top of the pyramid are fats, oils, and sweets, with the recommendation that those be used sparingly. Although this is a great improvement over the old depictions of the four food groups, most people cannot remain healthy on a diet which includes two to four servings daily of meat and two to three servings daily of dairy products.

Scientific Research Demands a Different Nutritional Plan

The 1992 USDA Food Guide Pyramid offers too little, too late. Responsible medical practitioners and scientists could not remain silent while yet another generation remained in darkness concerning health strategies. The new nutritional plan, first proposed on 8 April 1991, by the Physicians Committee for Responsible Medicine (PCRM) is called the New Four Food Groups. The program recommends that we consume a diet of grains, legumes, vegetables, and fruits. This group acknowledges the essential role of a high-fiber vegetarian diet in preventing and reversing degenerative disease. Dr. Denis Burkitt, Dr. T. Colin Campbell, and Dr. Dean Ornish are among the notable supporters of the New Four Food Groups. Dr. Burkitt is a medical pioneer whose research has documented the role of fiber in preventing degenerative disease. "His name and work are studied by every medical student in the world."[10] T. Colin Campbell, Ph.D., the Jacob Gould Schurman professor of nutritional biochemistry at Cornell University in Ithaca, New York, is the director of the China Diet Health Project, a study of more than sixty-five hundred Chinese living in sixty-five counties in China.[11] After studying the greatly varied regional eating habits of China, Dr. Campbell has concluded that the healthiest diet in China derives less than 10 percent of its protein from animal sources such as meat, milk, eggs, and cheese. The region which has the lowest risk of breast and colon cancer, diabetes, hypertension, and heart disease is also the region which eats mostly plant derived foods, such as rice, mushrooms, snow peas, bean sprouts, and bamboo shoots.[12] Dean Ornish's findings have been called "landmark research"[13] by Alexander Leaf, M.D., chairman of the Department of Preventative Medicine and Clinical Epidemiology at Harvard Medical School.

> Dr. Dean Ornish's internationally acclaimed scientific study, funded in part by the National Institutes of Health and based on thirteen years of research, has yielded astonishing conclusions: heart disease can often be halted or even reversed—without bypass surgery, angioplasty, or cholesterol-lowering drugs—simply by changing our life-style.[14]

The studies of Drs. Ornish and Campbell support a diet of grains, legumes and beans, fruits and vegetables. The Physicians Committee for Responsible Medicine does not recommend meat, fish, or chicken as a protein source, nor does the committee recommend the use of milk or milk products. Dean Ornish suggests the use of nonfat dairy products in moderation. Dr. Neal Barnard's *Food for Life* suggests a strictly vegan approach. He does *not* suggest nonfat dairy, but rather fruit sorbet or nondairy desserts. A vegan diet does not include meat, fish, chicken, eggs, or dairy.

We should carefully consider whether to eat meat, poultry, fish, eggs, and dairy in moderation or whether we should avoid those foods completely.

We need to evaluate the quantity and the quality of the meat, fish, and chicken which we consume.

Many Christians are unwilling to discuss the dangers of eating meat, fish, and chicken. But, if we look at cultures in which the people consume only 10 percent of their protein from animal sources, we see that the people have clearly benefited by eating meat, fish, and chicken in moderation. We may be accustomed to seeing platters of meat or individual servings of meat covering half a plate, but what is a "reasonable" portion?

As Christians, we need to address the issue of consuming too much meat. Is the "average American portion" a glutton's portion? Do our bodies need the amount of cholesterol and fat which we consume in the meat that we eat?

As Christians, we need to address the issue of consuming contaminated meat. Are we willing to eat meat which has up to sixteen times the amount of pesticides that we would get from an equivalent amount of grain or vegetables? If we cannot buy, or produce our own, meat that is safe, are we willing to abstain from eating meat?

As Christians, we need to address the issue of consuming contaminated fish. Are we willing to ingest PCBs, mercury, DDT, and chemical pollutants and pesticides which are present in 25 to 90 percent of the fish tested? Are we willing to expose ourselves to the bacterial contamination which is present in 40 percent of the fish at the supermarket counters? Are we willing to risk ingesting fish which have cancerous tumors? Do we need the cholesterol and fat which are present in fish?

As Christians, we need to address the issue of contaminated chicken. Are we willing to purchase chicken knowing that one in three packages of chicken contain live salmonella bacteria growing inside? Are we willing to purchase chicken from the supermarket knowing that federal regulations make it legal to sell salmonella-tainted chicken? Are we willing to consume chicken which we know has been raised in a crowded building, in the excrement of thousands of other birds? Are we willing to bring into our kitchens packages of chicken filled with water, blood, lymph, and feces?

High-fat Diets Increase the Level of Estrogens

Children are at risk as evidenced by the drop in the age of puberty. Women are at risk as evidenced by the increase in breast cancer.

> In 1840 the age of puberty in girls in Western countries was seventeen; today it is 12.5 years. In 1910, Americans got almost sixty percent of their calories from carbohydrates and about twenty percent from fat. By 1980, Americans consumed only about forty percent of their calories from carbohydrates and almost forty percent as fat.[15]

That simply means that as a nation we consume twice as much fat as our grandparents did. As a people, we are now fatter as a result. But, that is not the only problem. Meat, poultry, dairy products, and fried foods all cause an increase in the levels of estrogens in the blood. Diets low in fiber and high in fat allow the estrogens to remain in the digestive tract and become reabsorbed into the bloodstream. When a woman eats an increase in grains and vegetables, her estradiol level drops.[16] Dr. Neal Barnard cites Dr. Denis Burkitt's studies in Africa and Dr. T. Colin Campbell's research in China as further evidence that a low-fat diet keeps the age of puberty in girls higher (an average age of seventeen in rural China and rural Africa).[17] It is important for both boys and girls to consume a high-fiber, low-fat diet.

Dr. Dean Ornish recommends a vegetarian diet as the means of reducing a woman's blood estrogen level. He states that in Japan, where the consumption of animal fat is much lower, breast cancer is rare. However, he emphasizes that it is not because their genes are different:

> When Japanese women move to the United States and begin consuming a high-fat diet, they develop breast cancer at about the same rate as Americans—more than 400 percent higher than Japan. In part, this may be because a diet high in animal fats increases both the production and the biological activity of estrogens.[18]

Children's Fat-Laden Diet Causes Early Heart Disease

In September of 1993, the results of the largest autopsy study ever conducted on adolescents and young adults were released:

> Drawing on 1,532 autopsies of teen-agers and young adults who died from trauma in a dozen U.S. cities the study found that the coronary arteries of half bore the marks of early disease by the age of 19, while one hundred percent of adolescents had fatty patches in the aorta, the body's main artery.[19]

This is a far worse report than the study published over forty years ago revealing that most of the Americans killed in the Korean War had early signs of heart disease. The report about the American soldiers shocked most of the medical professionals at the time. Dr. Jack P. Strong of the Louisiana State University Medical Center and leader of the project, made these sobering observations:

> The take-home message of this report is that the earliest lesions are well established in practically all these subjects in this 15- to 34-year-old age group. The more advanced lesions begin to protrude into the blood vessel and narrow it beginning in the teens. By age 30 to 34 they are present in a rather

large proportion of the aortas and right coronary arteries.[20]

All of the American children who are consuming the standard American diet, high in fat, low in fiber, can be certain that there will be fatty deposits in their blood vessels by the end of their teen-age years. The article reporting Strong's study goes on to discuss cholesterol levels:

> A 1991 report from the National Heart, Lung and Blood Institute said the blood cholesterol levels of U.S. children and adolescents should be no higher than 170 milligrams per deciliter. Adults are considered to have high cholesterol if their level is above 240. The current average cholesterol level for all Americans is 205 milligrams, and the target for adults is an average level of 200 milligrams by the year 2000.[21]

Dr. Neal Barnard cites the Framington Heart Study as a more realistic approach to setting targets for cholesterol levels. No one in the thirty-five years of that study has had a heart attack whose blood cholesterol has been under 150. A lot of people who have a cholesterol level of 190 to 200 do have heart attacks.[22] We need to seek the ideal cholesterol level of 150, not 200!

Before we leave the issue of heart disease and the dangers of a high-fat diet, we need to ask ourselves what kind of a health strategy has been proven to reverse degenerative disease. Dr. Dean Ornish's program for reversing heart disease features dietary changes and lifestyle changes. The Reversal Diet in Dr. Ornish's program contains 10 percent dietary fat (mostly polyunsaturated and monounsaturated); 70 to 75 percent carbohydrate (primarily complex carbohydrates); and 15 to 20 percent protein. [23]

Here are Dr. Ornish's remarks about the Reversal Diet:

> The Reversal Diet is a very low-fat vegetarian diet, with no animal products except egg whites and nonfat dairy. This is what the patients in our study consumed, whose coronary heart disease began to reverse. I am convinced that this is the

world's healthiest diet for most adults, whether
or not they have heart disease.[24]

Dr. Ornish says that nonfat milk and nonfat yogurt
help to insure an adequate diet for those who do not eat
a varied diet. Separating the fat from the milk and egg
whites from the yoke, as Dr. Ornish recommends, is what
Annemarie Colbin calls "a reasonable approach from a
mechanistic nutritional viewpoint that holds protein in
high esteem and disparages fat."[25] Many others, this writer
included, disagree with the use of egg whites and nonfat
dairy as a means of insuring an adequate diet; a far better
plan is simply to eat a more varied diet. We can easily
obtain foods with sufficient protein, high fiber, low fat,
and vitamin B12 from plant sources. The Physicians Committee for Responsible Medicine does not recommend eggs
or dairy products. Dr. Neal Barnard insists that the "power
foods" are foods from plants and that they are the most
effective in preventing and curing all degenerative disease, including heart disease:

> The power foods are foods from plants. Vegetar-
> ians have a much better menu for the heart. Lacto-
> ovo-vegetarians (those who shun meats, poultry,
> and fish, but consume dairy products and eggs)
> do much better than those on lean meat diets,
> while pure vegetarians who steer clear of all ani-
> mal products do best of all.[26]

Dr. Barnard cites numerous studies comparing the
cholesterol levels and the rates of heart disease among
various vegetarian groups in the country. Clearly, the vegetarians have the lowest rates of coronary disease of any
group in the country; but among the vegetarians, vegans
(those who eat no eggs or dairy products) are the healthiest of all.[27]

It seems reasonable that if our bodies are in a weakened condition—for whatever reason—we should eat those
foods which will best enable us to achieve optimal health.
Some people will do well by avoiding meat and meat prod-

ucts only until they have achieved the health benefits they are seeking. Later, they may be able to maintain good health by consuming a maximum of 10 percent of their dietary fat from animal sources (red meat, fish, poultry, eggs, and dairy products).

The Problem with Milk

We talk to many mothers who have an uneasiness about milk, but they are haunted by their physicians' warnings not to deny children milk products. Gary and I heard the same warnings. Still, we fed our first two children only soy cheese and soy milk. Then, after the next two children got to pizza-eating age, we relaxed our standard and included dairy for pizza in our dietary regime. They also enjoyed milk at the homes of friends and grandparents and other relatives. We also switched from nondairy frozen desserts to the nonfat yogurt variety. We never stopped eating tofu. Each of our children has eaten it since birth. But, now we have gone from a little dairy to no dairy, and we are committed to staying dairy free! We use wonderful soy cheeses for pizza and sandwiches, and the children find the nondairy frozen desserts completely satisfying. Parents need to examine the evidence for themselves. I suggest purchasing the book, *Don't Drink Your Milk*, by Frank A. Oski, M.D. Dr. Oski is director of the Department of Pediatrics, at Johns Hopkins University School of Medicine and physician-in-chief at the Johns Hopkins Children's Center. Although Dr. Oski is not alone in recognizing the hazards of milk, his position at Johns Hopkins make him a credible resource for parents who find themselves at odds with the hometown pediatrician. Dairy products are not included in the New Four Food Groups and for many good reasons. Many common problems simply go away after milk and milk products are removed from the diet. Conditions associated with the consumption of cow's milk are asthma, allergies, strep throat, tonsillitis, ear infections, pimples, acne, and obesity. Dr. Neal Barnard's list of ten reasons for removing dairy from your diet is often summarized and quoted. We offer an abridged version of it here with the suggestion that the reader purchase and read *Food for Life*. The list is even more meaningful in context with the other chapters of Dr. Barnard's book.

Reasons Not to Drink Milk[28]

1. Milk is ineffective in preventing osteoporosis and slowing bone loss. Diets which are high in animal protein cause more calcium to be excreted.

2. Dairy products contribute cholesterol and fat to the diet. Studies show that the cardiovascular status of vegans is superior to that of lacto-ovo-vegetarians.

3. Comparisons of various countries shows a correlation between the use of dairy products and insulin dependent diabetes.

4. Numbers of people experience lactose intolerance, an acute reaction to milk which may include any or all of the following symptoms: cramps, bloating, intestinal gas, and diarrhea. (Among the lactose intolerant are: 70 to 90 percent of the blacks, Chinese, Japanese, Ashkenazi Jews, and Mediterraneans; and 25 percent of the Caucasian population.)

5. Milk is one of the most common food allergies. Respiratory problems, canker sores, skin conditions, and other subtle and not-so-subtle allergies can be caused by dairy products.

6. Dairy products frequently contain contaminants, from pesticides, chemicals, and drugs. One in every three cartons of milk contain some of the antibiotics that were fed to the cow. Twenty different antibiotics and thirty different drugs are legal for use in dairy cows. Even though farmers are prohibited from selling the milk of medicated cows, there is no regulatory system in place which can assure the consumer that farmers obey the rules.

7. Cow's milk is often the cause of colic in babies who are breastfed and whose mothers are drinking cow's milk. Babies who are fed cow's milk at birth frequently have colic.

8. Milk actually causes iron deficiency: first, because it has a low iron content and tends to replace iron-rich foods; and second, because milk can also cause the loss of blood from the intestinal tract, which over time reduces the body's iron stores. (Researchers speculate that bovine albumin, a protein present in milk, may elicit an immune reaction that leads to blood loss;[29] and third, dairy products interfere with the body's absorption of iron.)

9. Ovarian cancer is linked to dairy consumption and the problem is not solved by nonfat dairy products; the problem is with the milk sugar and not the fat. The problem arises when the consumption of dairy products exceeds the enzymes' capacity to break down galactose; a buildup of galactose occurs in the blood which may damage a woman's ovaries. Women who have low levels of these enzymes can have triple the risk of ovarian cancer if they consume dairy on a regular basis. Yogurt and cottage cheese present a greater threat because the bacteria used in their production actually increases the production of galactose from glucose.[30]

10. Populations that consume large amounts of dairy products have a much higher incidence of cataracts than do those who avoid dairy products. Again, the problem is not the milk fat, it is the milk sugar.

Those who insist on giving dairy to their young children would do well to provide them with the fresh, raw, unpasteurized milk from healthy, unmedicated goats. Certainly, when breast feeding is not possible, then goat's milk is the next best thing. In biblical times, goats were an important item in the pastoral wealth of the Near East. Goats' milk was preferred over any other. Proverbs 27:27 states that "there will be goats' milk enough for your food, for the food of your household, and sustenance for your maidens." At one time, I believed that yogurt and fermented milk (kafir and buttermilk) from goats ought to be included in an optimal diet. But, most of us have weakened our bodies by eating too much meat and cow's milk; by eating devitalized grain products; by eating an abundance of sugar and caffeine; and by consuming a variety of chemical contaminants through our water, air, and food supply. And, we can strengthen our weakened bodies most effectively by consuming grains, legumes, vegetables, and fruit. Research clearly indicates that most people are not achieving optimal health by consuming meat and dairy. If we are to regain our health, God's original plan (Gen. 1:29) is the best prescription.

Appreciate the Delicious Array of Foods which God has Provided

The Physician's Committee for Responsible Medicine recommends grains, vegetables, fruits, and legumes as the basis for an optimal diet. Sweeteners and oils are not included in their guidelines. However, in the recipe section of *Food for Life*, Dr. Barnard has included "oil-sprayed" pans and baking sheets and raw sugar. Also, olive oil is included in a recipe for Middle Eastern lentils and a delightful salad dressing recipe. Although I greatly admire the work of the Physicians Committee for Responsible Medicine, I believe that it is essential to include sweeteners and oils in any dietary guidelines. Some sweeteners and oils may be consumed in a dietary regime that builds optimal health. Consumers need to understand the differences in various sweeteners; the way in which they metabolize determines whether the sweeteners help us or harm us. And, the quantity of fat in our diets is not the only issue of importance. We must understand the differences in various types of oils and recognize the danger in many chemically processed oils. Also, nuts and seeds cannot be dismissed as totally hazardous and useless foods. They have a place in the diets of healthy children and adults. We deal with the question of who should avoid nuts and seeds in Step Five. Here, in Step Two, we have included *Sweeteners* and *Essential Fats* as the Fifth Food Group.

Five Essential Food Groups for Optimal Health and Nutrition

The vegetables which Daniel requested in Daniel 1:12 refer to "something sown," according to Bible dictionaries. It is likely that Daniel ate a variety of grains, legumes, vegetables, fruits, nuts, and seeds. Certainly, all of those foods were available in Genesis 1:29. As we discuss the benefits of these five food groups, we can easily understand why Daniel, Hananiah, Mishael, and Azariah were healthier than those who had been eating the king's choice food.

Group I–The Whole-Grain Group

Grains have been the main food for civilizations since ancient times. When we look at the amazing amount of energy required to build ancient cities and monuments, we must consider the grain which people consumed. Grains contain all of the nutrient groups which we require: carbohydrates, protein, fats, vitamins, minerals, and fiber. They are a wonderful source of B vitamins. Whole grains, unrefined, have three basic parts: the bran, the germ, and the endosperm. The complex sugars, or polysaccharides, which are abundant in grains include cellulose. These complex sugars are decomposed gradually by various enzymes in the mouth, stomach, pancreas, and intestines. They enter the bloodstream slowly, unlike the simple sugars (fruits and honey) and double sugars (cane sugar, sucrose, and milk sugar, lactose) which metabolized quickly. These intact grains (as opposed to grains which are ground into flour for bread and pasta) are the basis of an optimal diet. The protein content of the grain provides the building blocks that our body needs, and the complex carbohydrates assure a steady supply of energy for those who suffer from any blood sugar disorder. (Blood sugar disorders are epidemic and include numerous symptoms: weakness, fatigue, headaches, dizziness, depression, obesity—the list goes on.)

Bread, pasta, and cereal products should only be consumed if they are made from freshly milled flour. In Step

Three, we offer a complete discussion of milling and baking. But, even products made from freshly milled flour should not replace the intact grains our bodies require each day. Rice, millet, spelt, barley, and quinoa are our favorites for cooking. We mill hard white spring wheat, spelt, whole yellow corn, barley, and rice most frequently.

We must mention the question of cooking foods, as opposed to eating all of our foods raw. Many people who support the teaching of the natural hygienists believe that when we cook our food we destroy its nutritional value. They believe that when we eat cooked food we subject our bodies to a toxic residue which produces illness and shortens our lives. Many of these people eat no grain or beans because they require cooking. Others eat grains and beans, but limit their portions to 15 percent of their entire daily intake of food. They consume 85 percent of their food in the raw state.

In Step Four, we will discuss the importance of raw vegetable juices and an all-raw diet for those who are suffering from certain illnesses, but that kind of regime would not be a healthy one for many of us. Those of us who have suffered from hypoglycemia know that complex carbohydrates are a lifeline. While writing this book, I have not been eating any fruit. I eat bowls of raw vegetables—morning, noon, and night—and intact grain with every meal. This gives me a high level of energy. One piece of fruit, at times when I am working hard, causes me to feel tired. At night, and often at noon, I also eat beans or tofu. The proportions I use are five parts grain to one part beans or tofu.

Those who advocate a diet consisting only of raw fruits and raw vegetables believe that we can completely satisfy our protein requirement and all other nutritional requirements with raw fruits and vegetables alone. Medical and nutritional experts now disagree about the need to combine proteins. Some believe only vegetables and fruits are necessary; others believe grains and beans should be combined in one meal. It is important that we understand the great disagreement over important issues. It is a further reminder that we need to walk carefully and seek the Lord in all things. Here are four views regarding whether or not we need to combine foods in order to obtain all eight essential amino acids.

First is the view of Harvey and Marilyn Diamond whose book, *Fit for Life*, has popularized many of the teachings from the natural hygiene movement. They believe that protein obtained from vegetables and fruit is entirely sufficient to meet human needs.

> There are eight amino acids that the body must appropriate from outside sources, and although all fruits and vegetables contain most of the eight, there are many fruits and vegetables that contain all the amino acids not produced by the body: carrots, bananas, brussels sprouts, cabbage, cauliflower, corn, cucumbers, eggplant, kale, okra, peas, potatoes, summer squash, sweet potatoes, and tomatoes. Also all nuts, sunflower and sesame seeds, peanuts, and beans contain all eight as well.[32]

Second is Dr. Dean Ornish's advice concerning the need to combine protein.

> Unlike animal products, though, no single plant source contains all of the essential amino acids. Fortunately, though, plant-based foods contain the three critical amino acids in different proportions. By eating a variety of foods, you will obtain all of these necessary amino acids.
>
> Legumes are high in lysine but low in tryptophan and methionine. Grains are low in lysine but high in tryptophan and methionine. A meal of rice and beans, therefore, provides a complete protein, no different from the protein found in eggs and meat.
>
> You don't have to be a scientist or a nutritionist to combine foods properly. It's easy: just eat any grains and any legumes sometime during the same day.[33]

Dr. Ornish and the Diamonds would agree on this: Americans eat too much protein. Both the rich and the poor in this country eat at least twice as much protein as they need. Excess protein (from any source, plant or animal) can lead to bone demineralization and osteoporosis, as well as a number of degenerative diseases.

Now to make the discussion even more colorful, I will share a letter written to columnist Dr. Lamb and Dr. Lamb's reply. The column is entitled "Strict diet may affect amino acids" and the date is 24 January 1994.[34]

> Dear Dr. Lamb: I have given up red meat, pork and chicken for moral and ethical reasons. I eat eggs, some fish, beans and drink a little milk. Can I have a deficiency in protein and amino acids as well as iron?

> Dear Reader: You could. . . . Many ancient American civilizations survived in the past because they consumed both beans and corn. If you consume a sufficient quantity of fish that will also provide complete protein and prevent amino acid deficiencies. Iron requirements are more difficult to meet. Red meat is one of the best sources of iron. . . . You might also develop a B-12 deficiency.

We can understand why many people have been afraid to eliminate red meat from their diets. Eliminating fish, poultry, eggs, and milk is often unthinkable for people who have heard nothing but incorrect or incomplete information. Iron is a problem, but not the problem that Dr. Lamb suggests. Excess iron (most men have one thousand to two thousand extra milligrams in their bodies) causes heart disease, cancer, and premature aging. We now know that more people get in trouble from iron overload than iron deficiency. Our bodies are better able to limit the absorption of iron from vegetables, grains, and beans.[35] The meat and dairy industries offer advice along the lines that Dr. Lamb prescribes; but the Physicians Committee for Responsible Medicine recommends that we fulfill our protein, iron, and B12 requirements by eating foods from grain, bean, fruit, and vegetable sources.

I found a very simple explanation of the benefit in combining grains and beans. The author is an expert in dry legume cookery:

> Beans are about twenty to twenty-five percent protein, but they do not contain all of the essential amino acids and thus their protein is incomplete. However, complete protein can be formed by coupling beans with other protein sources. Grains, particularly rice, corn and wheat, are an excellent partner for the beans.[36]

One possible explanation for the very different views people have regarding how we are able to obtain essential protein is that individual human differences are often disregarded. People who are raised on low-protein diets, as in most of the world, are able to obtain the full nutritional value of plant food; their bodies work efficiently to accomplish this.

However, those of us who were raised on animal protein are often unable to obtain the full nutritional value of plant food when we first stop eating meat and meat products.

That means that the grains which have all eight essential amino acids (spelt and quinoa) serve us especially well. If by eating a small portion of beans with our grain dishes we are able to increase our strength and vitality, then we can be fairly certain that combining these nourishing plant foods is to our advantage. Finally, in both the natural hygiene healing system and the macrobiotic healing system people who are classified as "terminally ill" are often healed. Such healings have been well documented in both movements for decades. And yet, these healing systems are in direct opposition to each other. The natural hygienists advocate an all-raw diet and recommend large quantities of raw fruits. The macrobiotic teachers encourage 60 percent whole grains (intact), lightly cooked vegetables (20 to 30 percent), and no raw fruit. Both systems recognize important aspects of health and healing. Eliminating meat, fish, poultry, eggs, milk, spices, oil, sugar, and stimulants often allows our bodies to begin healing themselves. In the macrobiotic healing system, flour products are avoided when the body is in a weakened state. Although there is a deceptive teaching underlying both of those healing systems which implies that incorrect dietary practices are at the root of all or nearly all problems we might encounter, both systems grow out of a respect for the incredible way in which the human body heals itself. As Christians, we recognize that not only are we "fearfully and wonderfully made," but that the Lord Himself is our Great Physician.

The Seventh Day Adventists approach the matter of food choices quite differently. They focus on optimal foods and discourage their members from eating foods which do not build health, but within the Five Food Groups For Optimal Health which we have suggested here, they would impose few restrictions. A 1975 epidemiological study showed that Seventh Day Adventists in California have 72 percent less cancer of the bladder than the general population. Numerous studies show that the Seventh Day Adventists have significantly fewer deaths from cancer and other degenerative diseases than the general population. The church encourages members to avoid meat, poultry, fish, refined foods, alcohol, stimulants, and spices. And, although they favor whole grains, legumes, vegetables, fresh fruits, and nuts, they recognize the need for diversified dietary regimes. The Physicians Committee for Responsible Medicine clearly allows for diversity as well.

We can enjoy a wide variety of foods even when we restrict our diets in order to overcome weaknesses or illnesses. The number of "power foods"—foods which build strength and facilitate healing—is quite large. We discuss power foods in Step Four.

Group II—The Legume Group

Beans, lentils, and peas are part of this important group. Not only do beans have no cholesterol, studies have shown that beans actually lower cholesterol levels even when people are consuming high-fat diets.[37] Beans are rich in iron, high in fiber, low in fat, and low in calories. All beans are high in protein. They contain more soluble fiber per serving than oat bran. Beans contribute an abundance of B vitamins to our diets, as well as calcium, zinc, potassium, magnesium, and copper.

Beans have been considered essential to the diet since the beginning of recorded history. Ancient South American civilizations ate beans, according to archaeologists; remains of lentils have been found in ancient Egyptian tombs. Chinese and Indian cuisine have always featured beans. Throughout the ages, soybeans and mung beans have been an important part of the culture of the Orient. Today, we find that Mexicans have grown accustomed to kidney beans. And, Cubans relish black beans, red beans, pinto beans, and black-eyed peas are favorites in the southwestern United States.

In our home, we eat any and all beans that are available. Chickpeas (garbanzo beans) are one of our favorites. We eat them warm with grains or cold with vegetable and grain salads. When we puree garbanzos with sesame seeds, lemon juice, garlic cloves, salt and water, we have the Middle Eastern dish called hummus. This is a lovely spread to use with unleavened bread. Our children favor black beans seasoned only with tamari sauce.

Soy products such as tofu, tempeh, and miso are healthful additions to the diet—in moderation. Tofu is high in protein, but not actually a whole food. Whole cooked soybeans contain 28 percent more iron and 90 percent more fiber and B vitamins than tofu, plus vitamins A and C, which tofu lacks.[38] Miso is made by processing soybeans or cereal grains (such as barley, rice, and wheat) with sea salt for a period of one and one-half years through slow fermentation. Miso comes in a paste form and makes a delicious base for soup. Miso is an excellent source of B12. We eat miso soup with rice several evenings a week. It is a simple, satisfying, and delicious fast food. Tamari is the traditional, naturally made soy sauce. Chemically processed soy sauce is artificially made in a short period of time. Fermentation greatly increases the B12 content of foods.

Tempeh, a fermented soybean cake, offers from 1.5 to 6.3 micrograms per one hundred grams (3.5 ounces), the size of an average serving. When we eat fermented soy products, we do not need any additional supplementation of B12. Miso, in particular, also contains isoflavones; studies indicate that these substances protect women from breast cancer by inhibiting the growth of blood vessels which nourish solid tumors.

Beans make a significant contribution to the diet. We need only a small amount at one meal. An ideal serving would be from four to five parts grain to one part beans. By consuming the soluble fiber in beans, we can lower LDL (the "bad cholesterol") by as much as 24 percent. Beans are also useful in lowering blood pressure. Beans play a vital role in stabilizing blood sugar levels. Eating beans and grains together is extremely effective in the treatment and cure of adult-onset diabetes.

People often avoid beans because they have difficulty digesting them. Two starches found in beans, stachyose and raffinose, are not easily broken down by digestive enzymes. When they remain in the digestive tract, they come in contact with intestinal bacteria. When this bacteria breaks the starches down into carbon dioxide and hydrogen, flatulence results.[39]

The best solution is simply to begin consuming a small amount of beans at a time. If we eliminate refined foods and harmful products from our diet (see "Deceptive Foods" later in this chapter), our systems learn to tolerate beans. An expert in dry legume cookery suggests a method which she says "eliminates" the problem. Digesting beans has not been a problem for anyone in our household, but rather than give up eating beans I would use the following method of preparation:

Wash the beans and cover them with water.

Soak the beans all day.

Put them in the freezer and leave them all night. (This breaks down the starch molecules.)

Cook the beans with sea salt until almost tender.

Add six papaya tablets or two tablespoons of papaya granules.

The method which we use routinely in our house is this:

Wash and sort beans and cover them with purified water.

Soak the beans overnight in the crock pot.

Turn on the crock pot early in the morning.

Beans are ready in the early afternoon.

Add garlic, onions, and any herbs and spices two hours before beans are finished cooking in the crock pot.

Beans crush easily in our mouths when they have been cooked long enough (a simple test for tenderness). They are great for any meal in any season—hot bean dishes are satisfying in the winter, and cold bean dishes strengthen and invigorate us in the summer.

Group III—The Vegetable Group

In April of 1994, Newsweek magazine published an article entitled "Beyond Vitamins."[40] The popular press finally acknowledged what whole foods advocates have been saying for years: whole foods, especially fruits and vegetables, prevent disease. Phytochemicals are the compounds present in fruits and vegetables which fight disease. These amazing compounds have never been isolated because until recently scientists did not know that they existed. And yet, there are thousands of phytochemicals in every bite we take of a fruit or vegetable. Although cancer in particular is a disease with multiple processes, phytochemicals are apparently able to block each process.

A substance called sulforaphane—a phytochemical found in broccoli, cauliflower, kale, brussel sprouts, and turnips—prevents laboratory animals from getting cancer. When scientists added sulforaphane to human cells, they discovered that it boosted the synthesis of anti-cancer enzymes.[41] According to the research, cooking vegetables does not destroy sulforaphane.

A simple tomato has over ten thousand phytochemicals. They stimulate the activity of the enzymes inside our cells, enzymes which detoxify cancer-causing activity. Think of eating cauliflower to prevent breast cancer: cauliflower contains indole-3-carbinol, which "triggers enzymes that nudge the precursor to break down into a harmless form of estrogen rather than the form linked to breast cancer."[42] The key to all of this is enzyme activity. In Step Four, we discuss the healthy cell concept and explain enzyme activity. Once we have a vision of life at the cellular level, we see God's plan for health. The Lord has made provision for us with fruits and vegetables. Isolated supplements can never provide the benefit and protection which are available in whole foods.

Green leafy vegetables are among the most important foods in this group. We discuss them fully in Step Four. They are among the "power foods."

Group IV–The Fruit Group

Fruits are rich in vitamins, carbohydrates, and soluble fiber. Those who do not have any difficulty maintaining a stable blood sugar level can enjoy a greater quantity of fruit than those who struggle with hyperinsulinism or diabetes. Those who advocate a natural hygiene regime insist that fruit is the answer for those who suffer from hypoglycemia. Clearly, it is not. Metabolism and activity are sustained through the gradual decomposition of polysaccharide glucose. Polysaccharide glucose is the complex sugar found in grains and vegetables. Fruit is filled with nutrients and enzymes which are important and health building, but not all individuals can eat an all-fruit breakfast and/or lunch and maintain their health and stamina. People who have strong, active endocrine systems may do well with large amounts of both vegetables and fruit, while others who have weaker systems may need more protein.[43] Some nutritionists theorize that the activity of the adrenal gland and the pituitary gland determine which proportion of fruits, vegetables, beans, and grains best serve us.

Common sense tells us that there is life in fresh fruit. It is cooling, cleansing, and delicious. The research shows us that the thousands of phytochemicals which we obtain from fresh fruits and vegetables are essential for optimal health. Vegetable and fruit juices have a place (as we examine in Step Four) when we are cleansing our bodies, strengthening our bodies, or treating a disease.

The waxes that have been recognized as safe by the U.S. Food and Drug Administration make fruit and vegetables look shiny and fresh. They seal in moisture and prevent these products from shriveling. The wax—which is part of a marketing strategy, not a health strategy—is made of shellac, paraffin, palm oil, or synthetic resins. Some fungicides which are mixed with these waxes may increase the risk of cancer and other diseases. The only way to eliminate the wax is to peel the food. It will not wash off. Many nutritionists suggest three servings of fruit per day. Fruits are often the easiest and healthiest answer for snacks and desserts. But again, some adults and children will do better with a raw vegetable salad, a whole grain cookie sweetened with a grain sweetener, or a piece of bread made from freshly milled flour. Raw fruits and vegetables are alkaline, and we need a great amount of alkaline foods in our diet; but with that in mind, we need to be alert to the fact that each individual requires a different balance of grains, beans, vegetables, and fruits in order to achieve or maintain optimal health.

Group V—Complex Carbohydrate Sweeteners, Fruit Juice Concentrates, and Essential Fats and Oils

It is possible to make breads, muffins, cookies, and cakes which do not destroy our health. We can produce delicious baked goods *without* using table sugar, turbinado sugar, commercially sold fructose, honey, or maple syrup; none of which offer us any nutritional advantages. Honey and maple syrup, used in moderation, would be the best choices from that group. However, there are significantly healthier alternatives. We can learn a great deal from Oriental cuisine, which features many lightly sweetened desserts. Dried fruits and fruit juices make excellent sweeteners. Also, complex carbohydrate sweeteners offer an excellent alternative to the "natural" sweeteners such as honey and maple syrup.

Yinnie (rice) syrup is a sweet, thick syrup which is made from brown rice and barley. This sweetener is delicious in baked goods. It provides a healthful alternative for hypoglycemics and diabetics who enjoy bread and muffins. But, all of us benefit greatly by using this complex carbohydrate sweetener.

Barley malt syrup is a thick, dark brown sweetener made from barley. Like yinnie rice syrup, it is an important alternative to honey and maple syrup.

Fruit juice sweeteners, both the juices and the concentrates, offer benefits. Frozen apple juice concentrate is a very sweet solution for cakes, cookies, and muffins. Frozen orange juice concentrate is an alternative for those households where no one is sensitive to citrus.

Prune juice and prunes are most remarkable of all. Baking fat-free desserts is simple by using prunes. The California Prune Board has published the news that substituting prune puree for butter, margarine, or oil in baked goods can remove the fat by 75 to 90 percent. The big news is that prune puree makes it possible to enjoy 100 percent fat-free baked goods. Muffins are light and delicious *without* oil, eggs, or milk. Sorbitol, the naturally occurring compound in prunes, makes prunes an ideal fat substitute. It brings out the flavor of other ingredients.

Prune puree: 1 and ½ cups (8 ounces) of pitted prunes and 6 tablespoons of water in food processor or blender. Pulse on and off until prunes are finely chopped. Makes one cup.

The advantages of a diet that is free from sugar are well known. Sugar causes metabolic changes in the body which drain the body's reserve of B-complex vitamins, as well as minerals. Sugar stimulates a desire for more sugar and actually hinders a natural appetite for essential foods. Natural sweeteners do not upset the body's natural balance as greatly as sugar. Holidays and special occasions can be celebrated with a vast array of wholesome desserts.

Fats and Oils

Certain fatty acids are described as essential to the body because the body does not produce them. These polyunsaturated fats are liquid and remain that way. They are known as vitamin F. The sources of polyunsaturated fats are nuts, seeds, vegetables, walnut oil, fish, and soy beans. Fish which are frozen within four hours after a catch do not smell "fishy," a smell which indicates that the fatty acids have started to break down and have become rancid. Fish from cold, deep waters are the best source of the omega-3 fatty acids. Salmon, albacore tuna, Atlantic mackerel, and Atlantic herring are in this group.

Only expeller pressed or cold pressed oils should be used. But, we do not recommend using any of the polyunsaturated oils for seasoning, but rather extra virgin olive oil which is a monounsaturated fat. Heating oils produces free radicals. All cooking should be done using water or other liquids, never oil. Muffins, cakes, and cookies can be fat free. We compromise when we make yeast breads and flatbreads. We use two tablespoons of olive oil and lecithin. All yeast breads can be made without oil.

Fulfilling the Need for Essential Fatty Acids

Linoleic acid (LA) is an essential fatty acid because the body does not produce it. Alpha linolenic acid (LNA) is considered by some experts to be an essential fat because the body only makes some of the LNA it needs from LA. Both LA and LNA are among the more than fifty essential nutrients that the body cannot produce. Both of these essential fatty acids are necessary to maintain health. The average diet does not include foods which are rich in the omega-3 (LNA) components. The primary sources for omega-3 fatty acids are seeds and plants from cold climates, oils extracted from cold-water fish, and green leafy vegetables.

Foods that contain omega-3 oil go bad quickly. Therefore, it is difficult to obtain these nutrients from processed foods which have an extended shelf life.

The omega-3 and omega-6 oils are two essential fatty acids that together function in several important ways:[44]

• They form the membranes of each of the billions of cells in our bodies.

• They control the way cholesterol works in our system.

• They compose a great amount of the brain's active tissue.

• They are the only fats which become prostaglandins.

Prostaglandins play a vital role in regulating the functions of our vital systems: cardiovascular, immune, digestive, and reproductive. Prostaglandins control body heat and calorie burning, inflammation and healing, and the functioning of the brain.

Most of us are consuming sufficient quantities of omega-6 which is obtained from vegetable oils, but many of us are lacking in omega-3 oils. All dark green leafy vegetables contain large amounts of omega-3, but flaxseed has a higher content of omega-3 oil than any other food. Flaxseed contains twice as much as fish oil, and it is more stable. If we grind flaxseed, we need to consume it immediately because it goes rancid quickly. When we buy flaxseed oil, we must first be sure that it is dated; and then we must consume it before the expiration date. In order for flaxseed oil to be effective, it must be cold-pressed below forty degrees centigrade, unrefined, unfiltered, and nondeodorized. Because of these needs, mass processing methods are usually not acceptable.[45]

Dr. Johanna Budwig, a German Nobel Prize nominee, argues that many contemporary diseases are the result of fatty degeneration and essential fatty acid deficiencies.[46] As early as 1953, Dr. Budwig reported that she could change the yellow green protein substance in the blood of cancer patients into a red blood pigment or hemoglobin by giving those patients four ounces of nonfat cottage cheese and three tablespoons of fresh flax oil per day for three months. The Gerson Institute, well-known for its success in the treatment of cancer patients, now uses flax oil daily for their cancer patients.[47] A number of degenerative diseases are related to omega-3 deficiencies: heart attacks, arthritis, skin problems, immune system disorders, and mental illness.

There are many companies which produce and market flaxseed products. Listed here are those in the United States and Canada from whom we could obtain toll-free numbers:

Arrowhead Mills	1-800-858-4308 110 S. Lawton Street Hereford, TX 79045
Jarrow Formulas	1-800-334-9310 1824 S. Robertson Los Angeles, CA 90035
Nutri-Cology, Inc., Allergy Research Group	1-800-545-9960 400 Preda Street San Leandro, CA 94577
Omega Nutrition USA, Inc.	1-800-661-3529 Box 1979 Ferndale, WA 98248
Omega Nutrition	1-800-661-FLAX 8564 Frasier Street Vancouver, B.C., CANADA

During the two-year period in which I regained my health and lost all excess weight, I ate only the fats contained in grains, vegetables, legumes, salmon (omega-3 fatty acids), and extra virgin olive oil (a monounsaturated fat).

I never measured and never worried about fat grams. I ate a can of red salmon every day (I now use flaxseed oil instead). I used extra virgin olive oil on all of my vegetables and salads (and I still do). I became strong, energetic, and thin. I did not know about the benefits of flaxseed oil at that time. Flaxseed oil contains twice as much omega-3 fatty acids as fish oil and has none of the environmental pollutants which we find in fish oil.

It is important to take note of this point: While I consume a great deal of omega-3 fatty acids and a great deal of extra virgin olive oil, I do not consume any other oils or any animal fat. When I consume grains, vegetables, and beans, I eat the fats which are present in those whole foods.

Nuts and seeds—in moderation—are a good source of fat for healthy adults and children who tolerate them. Many people cannot tolerate them, a subject which we discuss in Step Four. While my husband and children enjoy them occasionally, I do not eat nuts and seeds. The research supports a dietary regime which includes beneficial fats. Some fats are essential for good health.

Extra Virgin Olive Oil

In a quest to discover health secrets from around the world, scientists have found one place where people consume fatty diets and, yet, have virtually no coronary heart disease. That place is the island of Crete where the traditional diet of the residents derives 35 to 40 percent of its calories from fat. For generations, the people there have consumed olive oil in lavish quantities: with cooked vegetables, with pasta dishes, in sauces, as a spread for bread. The native diet is also low in meat, and rich in vegetables, fruits, and grain.

Scientists studying cardiovascular disease suspect that monounsaturated fat, the kind in olive oil, may reduce the body's level of "bad cholesterol" (LDL—Low-Density Lipoproteins) and actually boost the levels of "good cholesterol" (HDL—High-Density Lipoproteins). Critics charge that the results achieved in Crete have more to do with the grains, fruits, and vegetables than with the olive oil. Others correctly point out that the unrefined oil used by the Greek farmers is quite different than the olive oil on the super-market shelves.

Only extra virgin olive oil should be consumed. The unrefined extra virgin olive oil available through natural foods suppliers is obtained from olives without undergo-ing chemical processes, only washing, sedimentation, and filtering.

Other Monounsaturated Fats

These fats are found in several foods, but not all of them are beneficial to the body. Olive oil, canola oil, and peanut oil all have monounsaturated fat. Canola oil has 5 percent erucic acid which affects many organs in the body. Peanut oil, like peanuts, is often contaminated by aflatox-ins. These aflatoxins may cause liver cancer. Other studies indicate that peanut oil appears to promote arteriosclero-sis. Avocados are an excellent food. One study showed that women who supplemented their otherwise low-fat diets with avocado lowered their cholesterol levels, maintained a high HDL level, and stayed with their diet longer than those who were on the standard low-fat regime.[48] I have encouraged women to include extra virgin olive oil in their low-fat diets. They are amazed that the cravings for sweets and fats cease, and they begin losing weight. Avocados work in the same way. The monounsaturated fats probably work in numerous ways which we have yet to discover. Those of us who have eaten these fats and have grown stronger and thinner know that they are important foods.

The Advantages of Nuts

Pecans, cashews, almonds, and hazelnuts are all rich in monounsaturated fats.

Nuts contain protease inhibitors which block cancer in test animals. They are also rich in polyphenols, chemicals which hinder the growth of cancer in animals. Peanuts are not nuts. They are actually legumes, and they are often contaminated with a mold called aflatoxin, which is a car-cinogen.

Deceptive Foods

> When you sit down to dine with a ruler
> Consider carefully what is before you;
> And put a knife to your throat,
> If you are a man of great appetite.
> Do not desire his delicacies,
> For it is deceptive food.
>
> —Proverbs 1:1–3

Deceptive foods often look appealing, tantalizing, and even nourishing, but they are lacking in the essential fiber, nutrients, and/or healthful fats which whole foods contain. Now that we have discussed what foods we should eat and why, it is easier to understand what not to eat. Deceptive foods bring death to the cells in our bodies. Here are the categories of foods to avoid: life-threatening fats; devitalized flour products; sugar and artificial sweeteners; soft drinks and caffeine; and salt.

Life-threatening Fats

Animal products: All animal products contain cholesterol. Dr. Neal Barnard tells us that:

> Every 100 mg. of cholesterol you eat in your daily routine adds roughly five points to your cholesterol level. (Everyone is different and this number is average.) In practical terms, 100 mg. of cholesterol is four ounces of beef, or four ounces of chicken, or half an egg, or three cups of milk.[49]

All animal products contain saturated fats. The fat molecule of the saturated fat is completely covered with hydrogen atoms. Saturated fats stimulate the liver to make more cholesterol, while polyunsaturated fats and monounsaturated fats do not. We can recognize saturated fats because they are solid at room temperature. Often consumers believe that they can avoid saturated fats by trimming the strips of fat off the meat and chicken. In the leanest cuts of beef, about 30 percent of the calories are from fat. In the leanest chicken, the figure is about 20 percent.[50]

Dr. Barnard uses the McDonald's McLean Deluxe Burger as an example of the deception that is prevalent in the marketplace. The company introduced the McLean Deluxe Burger with the announcement that it was 91 percent fat free. They had measured the fat content by weight. If we analyze the McLean Deluxe Burger patty itself, by the percentage of calories—the way that scientists and dietitians do—we find that the patty is 49 percent fat. If we add in the bun and the topping, we bring the number down to 29 percent fat. The 9 percent computation is simply not true.

We do not have to be a mathematician to determine whether the meat we are eating is "low-fat." Meat is not part of a "low-fat" regime.

Commercially Processed Vegetable Oils: These have been extracted with chemical solvents, degummed, bleached, refined, heated, and deodorized. The refining process removes the free fatty acids from the oil. Degumming removes nutrients such as chlorophyll, calcium, magnesium, iron, and copper. Synthetic antioxidants are frequently added to the supermarket oils. In order to deodorize oils, manufacturers expose the oils to extreme temperatures, 240–270 degrees. Unlike the healthy "cold processed" oil, these refined oils have removed that which is good and added that which is detrimental to our bodies. Coconut and palm kernel oils are just as high in saturated fat as animal fat, and yet they are classified as vegetable oil. Avoid them always. For your health, learn to love extra virgin, unrefined, cold pressed olive oil. Cook foods in water and other liquids, not oils!

Hardened Oils (Margarine and Shortening): For many years consumers denied themselves butter and used margarine in order to prevent coronary heart disease and other diseases. Vegetable oils are hardened by a process called hydrogenation. These oils increase serum cholesterol just as the saturated fats do. When manufacturers convert vegetable oils into shortening and margarine which are solid or semi-solid at room temperature, trans-fatty acids are formed in the process. These trans fats are anti-nutrients. They block the development of prostaglandins, hormone-like substances that are vital in regulating not only the cardiovascular system, but the reproductive system, the central nervous system, and the immune system.[51]

Hydrogenated oils, like margarine, not only clog the arteries, they are linked with tumor growth. But, the way in which trans-fatty acids block the development of pros-taglandins may be the most serious problem of all. Some researchers actually believe that the onset of any disease is due to a prostaglandin imbalance.

Liquid soybean oil is only 15 percent saturated fat; but when it is partially hydrogenated—a process used to make shortening like Crisco—the fat is increased to 25 percent. These trans-fatty acids are almost impossible for our bodies to eliminate.

The message is clear. Hydrogenating fat destroys the essential fatty acids. By eliminating the good (essential fatty acids) and adding the bad (trans-fatty acids), manufacturers give us a product which is now known to be hazardous to our health. Not only should we eliminate this deceptive food, we must make certain that we include the essential fatty acids, especially fresh flaxseed oil, in our diets to prevent and cure disease.

Unwholesome flour products (often referred to as "whole grain products" by bread, cereal, and pasta manufacturers)

The nutrients and the fiber found in freshly milled flour are an important part of the prevention and treatment of a number of common illnesses, among them are coronary heart disease, colon cancer, appendicitis, gall-stones, diverticular disease, diabetes, breast cancer, and hemorrhoids. Commercially milled and processed flour offers nothing at all which supports life.

When we mill flour at home, it is necessary to bake with it immediately or freeze it. If we leave it on the counter for even a few hours, the wheat germ and the wheat germ oil begin to deteriorate. Instead of a fresh, sweet smell, the product acquires a foul odor. Grains, as long as they are in their protective covering, can be stored for years. But once the bran is removed, the deterioration begins. When we buy bread, baked goods, cereals, pasta—anything made from grain in the supermarket—we are purchasing a devitalized product. Commercial millers remove 30 percent of the wheat kernel (and the most nutritious part of the grain) in order to make white flour. Why? The wheat germ and the wheat germ oil are the most nutritious parts, and they are also the quickest to spoil. Although 90 percent of the nutritional value of the wheat berry is in the wheat germ and the wheat germ oil, that is the portion which is removed from commercially ground flour. All of the "whole grains" in the supermarket are lifeless. We can usually find authentic brown rice in the supermarket, but other grains are seldom there. Most people have never seen a wheat berry or a kernel of spelt, quinoa, or millet.

Products made from white flour are deadly. Thousands of products in the supermarket are filled with unwholesome flour, table sugar, and fat. Most of the products which claim to be "whole-grain" are not "whole-grain" products at all. The only life-giving whole-grain products are the intact grains: (1) kernels of rice, millet, spelt, and barley; (2) cereals made from grains which are freshly flaked; (3) baked goods and cereals made with freshly milled flour. Breads, cereals, and baked goods, made from commercially milled flour are not life-giving products. Unless health food stores sell freshly milled flour and products made with freshly milled flour, their flour and flour products are equally harmful; devitalized flour does not become desirable simply because it has no pesticides. Bread is "the staff of life" if it is the real thing. Without wheat germ and wheat germ oil, it is just a deceptive food. In Step Three, we will discuss this important topic more fully.

Sugar and Artificial Sweeteners

Sugar

Making a case against sugar is beyond the scope of this book. Also, two wonderful books have been available for years, and I recommend them to everyone: *Sweet and Dangerous* by Peter Yudkin, M.D.,[52] and *Body, Mind, and Sugar* by E.M. Abrahamson, M.D., and A.W. Pezet.[53]

Dr. Yudkin, renowned physician, biochemist, and researcher, offers his pioneering studies about sugar. He explains why sugar is a health hazard to everyone. Dr. Yudkin presents a scientific case against sugar as the principle cause of numerous degenerative diseases.

Abrahamson and Pezet look at the relationship between fatigue, hay fever, ulcers, neurosis, alcoholism, migraine, insomnia, allergies, rheumatoid arthritis, epilepsy, depression, and the food people eat every day.

It is impossible to overstate the dangers of sugar. We accept this addiction as a part of life. Dr. Mary Ruth Swope, a sensitive and caring educator, nutritionist, and Christian, speaks plainly about sugar: "Sugar is a drug. Ten teaspoonfuls immobilize the immune system by thirty-three percent. Thirty teaspoonfuls shut down the system for a whole day."[54]

The average American consumes over two pounds of sugar a week. Manufacturers depend upon sugar to make their products appealing to the consumer; it is their most important additive.

In Step Three, we discuss advanced food dehydration. Dried fruits are rich in nutrients and are also delightfully sweet. There are simple, delicious, and healthy alternatives to sugar.

The best sweeteners are barley malt syrup, brown rice syrup, dried fruits, fruit juices, and fruit juice concentrates. If we avoid processed foods, we needn't worry about all of the different names for sugar. There are many:[55]

barley malt	grape sweetener
date sugar	herbal sweetener
beet sugar	polydextrose
blackstrap molasses	high fructose corn syrup
dextrin	honey
brown sugar	sorbitol
dextrose	invert sugar
cane sugar	sorghum

fructose	lactose
caramel	sucanat
fruit fructose	maltose
corn fructose	sucrose
glucose	manitol
corn sweetener	sugar
grape sugar	maple syrup
corn syrup	turbinado
raw sugar	molasses

Three proverbs comment on the role of honey in our diets and assure us that with His wisdom we will know how much "honey" is enough. This advice concerning honey would apply to all natural sweeteners.

> My son, eat honey, for it is good,
> Yes, the honey from the comb is sweet to your taste;
> Know that wisdom is thus for your soul;
> If you find it, then there will be a future,
> And your hope will not be cut off. (Prov. 24:13–14)

> Have you found honey? Eat only what you need,
> Lest you have it in excess and vomit it. (Prov. 25:16)

> It is not good to eat much honey. (Prov. 25:27)

Artificial Sweeteners

Acesulfame-K, aspartame, and saccharin are all health hazards. These sweeteners do not cause the same problems that sugar causes; they create new health risks. Consumer groups charge that acesulfame causes tumors in rats. The FDA approved this artificial sweetener in 1988. Aspartame is sold under the brand names Equal and NutraSweet. Numerous groups and individuals have objected to the FDA's approval of this artificial sweetener, because it poses a health hazard to children. Critics of all ages charge that the product causes headaches, dizziness, and seizures. Saccharin has been widely available for nearly a century. Studies have linked saccharin and bladder tumors in rats. The FDA proposed a ban, but the product remained on the market as a result of a consumer outcry in support of the product.

> Aspartame—sold under the brand names, NutraSweet and Equal—is composed of three molecules: phenylaline, aspartic acid and methyl alcohol. Methyl alcohol is a human specific, highly toxic poison. Furthermore, methyl alcohol is converted into formaldehyde and formic acid, both of which are carcinogenic because of their toxic effect on the immune system.[56]

Soft Drinks and Caffeine

Dr. Mary Ruth Swope has written a short paper entitled, "Why I Don't Drink Soft Drinks (And Wish You Didn't)." I have her permission to quote freely from that paper. What follows is an abridged version of her comments. I also share her research and a collection of testimonies by various experts in the field of health and nutrition. Dr. Swope is hopeful that multitudes of people will come to realize the danger in consuming soft drinks and find the will to stop consuming them. She also warns us about the danger in consuming any beverages which contain caffeine.

Disease flourishes in an acid pH, and cola type drinks are acid.

> All kinds of soft drink are very acidic, especially colas. In order to neutralize a glass of cola, it takes thirty-two glasses of high pH alkaline water.[57]

> If we could get our cells to maintain a normal pH (slightly alkaline), cancer could not grow in our bodies.[58]

Certain soft drinks may promote the development of cancer.

> Cancer is like a plant cell; it can't live in an oxygen-rich environment. Cola drinks make our bodies poor in oxygen. Cancer is the second cause of death in

America. The average American is consuming eight hundred or more soft drinks annually.[59]

The phosphoric acid in soft drinks affects the bones in our bodies. Dr. Swope challenges readers to pour cola over an extracted baby tooth or a ten-penny nail; either one will totally dissolve within a few days.

> A government warning was once issued to the manufacturer of a certain world-famous refreshing soft drink for its suspected effect on the bones of children because of the large amount of phosphoric acid contained in it.[60]

> Rats, well fed but given nothing to drink except cola beverages, after six months had their molar teeth dissolved down to the gum line. When Dr. McCay reported years ago the rat experiments before the Delaney hearings on chemicals in foods, a lawmaker reminded him that the soft drink industry represented huge economic investments.[61]

Soft drinks also damage the kidneys. As we get older our kidneys are less able to excrete phosphorus, causing a depletion of vital calcium. When soft drinks interact with antacids, they can cause kidney damage.Coffee, tea, and soft drinks all offer the drug caffeine. No matter how many caffeine drinks a day a person consumes, the habit is socially acceptable. Dr. Mary Ruth Swope has this to say about the gravity of the situation:

> Caffeine is a member of the same alkaloid group of chemicals as morphine, nicotine, cocaine, purines and strychnine. These alkaloids all have one thing in common: they are addictive. . . . Coffee is a drug and it acts as a stimulant to the nervous system. Soft drinks, including the cola and pepper-type drinks that have caffeine in them, are the most popular beverages in America today. Coffee is second.[62]

> In the amounts presently being consumed, it can cause insomnia, nervousness, irritability, anxiety, and

disturbances in the heart rate and rhythm. Cola and pepper-type drinks account for eighty to ninety percent of the caffeine added to foods today. Its long term effects on people are not clearly known.[63]

Salt

Salt is a major cause of high blood pressure in this country. When salt is overused it can cause a severe kidney disease called nephritis. Those who daily consume products which stress the kidneys—alcohol, tea, coffee, soft drinks, supplements, and salt—risk damaging their kidneys.

All salt is not the same. Some nutritionists recommend coarse ground sea salt. It can be used in a salt grinder or ground in a small, inexpensive electric mill.

Dr. Yoshihide Hagiwara, M.D., discusses the acid and alkaline balance in our bodies. He says that the consumption of reagent grade manufactured salt instead of the natural sea salt man used to use is one of the causes of an acid alkaline imbalance.[64]

Modern table salt has been refined so that many of the trace minerals found in natural sea salt are missing. Table salt is, of course, nearly 100 percent sodium chloride.

Table salt in combination with animal fat, sugar, caffeine, commercially milled flour, and soft drinks can in fact accelerate degenerative disease. If coarse ground sea salt is used moderately in a diet of whole grains, beans, fruits, and vegetables, there is considerably less danger to the kidneys. Both fresh herbs and dehydrated herbs enable us to be satisfied with far less salt. We can learn to appreciate the delightful flavor of many herbs and spices as well.

Locate Reliable Whole Foods Suppliers

Often health food stores do not have the produce, grains, and variety of foods we may require. Or, we sometimes find that these specialty stores must charge higher prices than we are willing to pay. However, there are wonderful exceptions across the country. We've worked closely with many proprietors who operate their businesses like old-time general stores; they offer discounts for volume purchases and delight in developing personal relationships with their customers.

Cooperative Warehouses are the answer for most of us who want to purchase healthful food in bulk at wholesale prices. We have been members of large "buying clubs" and we have organized a number of small groups (three or four families). Recently, two other women and myself organized a group. Each month, one of us collects the orders and calls them in. The truck comes to the house we designate. We meet and divide the order. Cooperative Warehouses have varied minimum requirements. If the minimum purchase requirement is high, then buying clubs must acquire a sufficient number of members to meet the monthly requirement. Small minimum requirements allow small groups to operate, and small groups simply require less time and energy than large groups do. These warehouses offer catalogues which make shopping convenient. Often local groups with common interests find it pleasant to get together to meet a common need. Home educators and church groups who are already supporting one another find this a meaningful way to share in the routine business of one another's lives. Other people form cooperative buying clubs based on a common desire to promote an interest in whole foods and whole foods cuisine.

No matter what Cooperative Warehouse we buy from, we all need to have a source for superior quality OCIA (Organic Crop Improvement Association) certified grains. We have worked with brokers and grain suppliers all across the United States and Canada; we now buy our grain from a grain specialist who deals directly with OCIA farmers. He never purchases the wheat before his wife bakes with a sample batch—no matter what the lab tests indicate. This family offers OCIA certified organic grains, the finest we have ever had. Their current organic grain supply includes: hard red winter wheat, hard white winter wheat, hard white spring wheat, and spelt. These grains bake beautifully. Our loaves of bread are high and fluffy. They operate their business from their small farm in Inman, South Carolina. We will furnish three useful items if you contact us: 1) their current price sheet with an ever-expanding assortment of grains, beans, nuts, and seeds; 2) an information sheet explaining the standards of OCIA (OCIA certified products are among the purest food products available in the United States); and 3) a list of grain suppliers across the United States who offer a wide assortment of products and services. If this wonderful Christian family cannot serve you, we will help you find someone who can. For all three pieces of information simply send a stamped, self-addressed envelope to the address listed below.

Healthy Living
P.O. Box 889
Columbus, NC 28722

Cooperative Listings

Serving the Northeastern United States:

E & S Sales
1235 North State Road 5
Shispshewana, IN 46565

Northeast Co-Op
POB 8188
Brattleboro, VT 05304

Clear-Eye Natural Foods
302 Rt. 89 Southeratives
Savanah, NY 13146-9790

Federation of Ohio River
Cooperatives
320 East Outerbelt Street
Columbus, OH 43213-1597

Associated Buyers
POB 207
Somersworth, NH 03878
603-692-6101

Dutch Valley Bulk Food
Distributors
Meyerstown, PA 17067
(Christian Company)
1-800-468-2963

Serving the Southeastern United States:

Friendship Buying Club
Rt. 2, Box 66A
Pleasant Shade, TN 37145

Serving: FL, AL, GA, NC, SC

Orange Blossom Cooperative Warehouse
1601 NW 55th Place
Gainesville, FL 32613-4159
1-800-372-7061

Serving: TX, LA, OK, MS, MO, AR, KS, AL, GA

Ozark Co-Op Warehouse
Box 1528
Fayetteville, AR 72702
1-501-521-4920

Serving: AZ, NM, parts of TX, CO, UT, NV, CA

Tucson Cooperative Warehouse
350 South Toole Ave
Tucson, AZ 85701
1-602-884-9951

Serving: AZ, CA, CO, ID, MT, NV, NM, OR, UT, WA, WY
(will ship containers to AK and HI)

Mountain Peoples Warehouse
110 Springhill Drive
Grass Valley, CA 95945
1-916-273-9531
1-800-833-9531

Serving: IA, IL, KN, KS, MI, MN, MO, NE, SD, WI, WY

Blooming Prairie Warehouse, Inc.
2340 Heinz Road
Iowa City, IA 52240
Member Services Department
1-319-337-6448

Serving: WA, OR, ID, NW corner of Montana
(other surrounding states may inquire)

Azure Standard
79709 Dufur Valley Road
Dufur, OR 97021
1-503-467-2230

Serving: WA, ID, OR

Nutrasource
POB 81106
4005 Sixth Avenue South
Seattle, WA 98108
1-206-467-7190;
In-state toll-free 1-800-762-0211;
Out-of-state toll-free 1-800-33-NUTRA

Serving: all across the United States

Walton Feed, Inc.
135 North 10th
P.O. Box 307
Montpelier, ID 83254
1-800-847-0465 or 1-208-847-0465

Stock the Pantry with Foods for Life

None of us can accomplish the tasks that God requires us to do without an obedient heart. Again and again we see that if we are obedient, He will give us the time, talent, and equipment to do the job. In the spirit of Titus, chapter two, young women are to "be sensible, pure, workers at home, kind" (Titus 2:5); and yet, even among professing Christians, the home is often no more than a way station. Clearly, God intended for the home to be a place where we nurture one another. Home is the place where we learn and practice the skills which equip us for life. Preparing food is an essential part of nurturing. As wives and mothers who seek to obey the Lord and to walk in the light of His Word, we are not free to decide that the kitchen is not the place for us. I meet many Christian women—young and old—who want to escape as much food preparation as possible. Those who have servants to do essential tasks, while they do other chores which God has called them to do, can still take care of their households properly. Many of my friends on the mission field are in that situation. Others I know simply have the income to hire the help they need. But, whether we have no children and many servants (as is the case of a dear friend of mine), or many children and no servants (as is the case of many, many friends of mine), we need to heed the call of Proverbs 31 and provide for our households. What is more important than taking the time to stay well and to stay alive! We must take time to read the Bible that we may "live and keep Thy word"; and we must take time to prepare, serve, and consume the foods which He has provided that we may walk in His health and healing. I urge every child and every woman who knows the Lord to seek His face in this most important matter of learning essential tasks. Whether we are eight or eighty, we are indeed blessed if we have the physical strength and the mental ability to take care of ourselves and those we love. All male children should learn every aspect of food preparation simply because both men and women are called to care for one another at different times. If a household shuts down simply because the wife and mother is away or ill, that indicates that the husband and children need training in order be the servants we are all called to be. It is encouraging to think of our Lord making provisions for His disciples by the Sea of Galilee. First, He made it possible for them to catch the fish which they had been unable to catch; then, as their Servant, He prepared a meal for them there by the sea:

> And so when they got out upon the land, they saw a charcoal fire already laid, and fish placed on it, and bread. Jesus said to them, "Bring some of the fish which you have now caught." Simon Peter went up, and drew the net to land, full of large fish, a hundred and fifty-three and although there were so many, the net was not torn. Jesus said to them, "Come and have breakfast." (John 21:9–12)

Four Pantries Which Accommodate Our Food Storage Needs:

The Dry Pantry

Grains: barley, short grain brown rice, long grain brown rice, spelt, millet, quinoa, hard red spring wheat, hard white spring wheat, whole yellow corn, hopi blue corn, kamut, amaranth, oats groats, popping corn.

We store our grains in twenty-five and forty-five pound buckets in a storage room at the rear of our garage. We keep some grains and beans in glass containers in the kitchen for convenience.

(Notice that there are no flours or cereals in the dry pantry. Since all freshly milled flour or freshly flaked cereal must be used immediately or stored in the freezer, flours and cereals are listed in the freezer pantry. Also, breads and pasta which cannot be consumed within two days from the time of milling and baking are also stored in the freezer pantry.)

Baked Goods: breads, rolls, muffins, cookies, to be consumed within three days from milling and baking.

Beans: adzuki, black beans, garbanzos, kidney beans, lentils, navy beans, pinto beans, red beans, soy beans, split peas.

Vegetables and Herbs:

Fresh: potatoes (Irish and sweet), squash (all varieties), garlic bulbs (always on hand), peppermint leaves.

Canned: organic tomato sauce, organic tomato paste, organic tomato puree.

Dehydrated: These may be stored as vegetable roll-ups, vegetable chips, or powdered for use as seasonings in many recipes: asparagus, beans, beets, broccoli, brussels sprouts, cabbage, carrots, cauliflower, celery, corn, cucumbers, eggplant, kohlrabi, lettuce, lima beans, mushrooms, okra, onions, parsnips, peas, peppers, potatoes, pumpkin, radishes, spinach, squash, swiss chard, tomatoes, yams, zucchini. (Vegetables from the garden or from the market can be easily dehydrated and stored for use throughout the year.)

Fruits:

Fresh: bananas

Canned: pumpkin

Dehydrated: These may be stored as fruit leathers, fruit chips, or in powdered form to be used as sweeteners:

apples, apricots, bananas, blueberries, cherries, citrus rinds, coconut, cranberries, dates, figs, grapes, melons, nectarines, papaya, peaches, pears, pineapple, plums, raspberries, rhubarb, strawberries.

Bottled Fruit Juice: prune juice for use in baking bread, muffins, cookies, and cakes.

Powdered Drinks: carob powder, dry soy milk powder, whole foods concentrates (Barleygreen, Just Carrots, RediBeets).

Baking Supplies: Dough Enhancer (all natural ingredients including citric acid which preserves bread and improves its texture), Pro Wheat Gluten (helpful when baking with nonglutinous grains and beans), Watkins Baking Powder (contains no aluminum), SAF instant yeast (freeze after opening).

Nuts and Seeds: walnuts, pecans, and almonds for nut butters.

Oil: extra virgin olive oil.

Miscellaneous: agar (vegetable gelatin), arrowroot flour, and coarse ground sea salt.

The Condiment Pantry

Sweeteners: fruit-only jellies and butters, molasses and honey (for baking), barley malt syrup (for baking).

Herbs and Spices: Many of the vegan (no meat, fish, chicken, eggs, or dairy) cookbooks we recommend are written by Seventh Day Adventists, who do not use spices. I include spices here because I frequently cook and bake with them. My husband uses pepper occasionally, and I often bake with cinnamon. Rice and grain dishes offer endless variety when they are seasoned with the herbs and spices listed below. Although I do not consume spices personally, I offer them to my family and to our friends and guests who enjoy them.

We buy all of our herbs and spices from Watkins. They are delivered directly to our home. This company is over 125 years old. Watkins has stringent quality control standards, and the spices are protected against insect infestation, hazardous chemicals, and direct sunlight. They are free of fillers and waste particles which are common in other spices we have used. The herbs and spices arrive in tightly sealed glass bottles to insure freshness. And, they are popularly priced. We no longer buy any spices in bulk from cooperative warehouses and never from the supermarket. I discovered Watkins pepper and cinnamon while looking for something in a friend's kitchen cabinet. When I smelled her spices, I knew that I needed to restock our condiment pantry. Watkins representatives allow customers to smell, touch, and taste the products. Herbs and spices are an important part of food preparation; enjoying the very best condiments available won't cost anymore than purchasing grossly inferior ones.

Pepper Blends: black pepper, Cajun pepper, cracked pepper, dijon pepper, herb pepper, Italian pepper, lemon pepper, Mexican pepper.

Pepper Corns: garlic peppercorn blend, royal peppercorn blend.

Gourmet Seasoning Blends: allspice, basil, celery seed, cilantro, cinnamon, cloves (ground), cumin, curry powder, dill weed, garlic flakes, garlic granules, ginger, Herbes de Provence, Italian seasoning, Mexican oregano, minced green onion, mustard (dry), nutmeg, onion powder granules, oregano, paprika, parsley, rosemary, tarragon, thyme.

Flavorings: Pure vanilla extract and pure almond extract.

The Refrigerator Pantry

Tofu, miso paste, tamari soy sauce, raw unfiltered apple cider vinegar.

Fruits: Apples, lemons, oranges, berries, others in season, locally grown grapes in season.

Vegetables: Carrots, cauliflower, cabbage (purple and green), scallions, yellow onions, white onions, purple onions, broccoli, celery, kale, collards, parsley, watercress, romaine lettuce, tomatoes.

Prepared Foods: Spelt, rice, beans. (We usually have two cooked grains and one type of cooked beans in the refrigerator for quick meal preparation.)

Jams and Jellies, Nut Butters and Spreads: Jams and jellies sweetened only with fruit, almond butter, pecan butter, walnut butter, Spectrum Spread (non-hydrogenated, no trans-fatty acids, nondairy cholesterol free—made from a patented process mixing canola oil and water).

Oils: Flaxseed oil (must be refrigerated and used before the expiration date), unrefined extra virgin olive oil (should be refrigerated).

The Freezer Pantry

Fruit Juice Concentrates: Apple juice, orange juice (for baking).

Whole Grain Products: (made from freshly milled grains or freshly flaked grains):

Pizza dough (already rolled out), trays of cinnamon rolls (ready to bake), pie crusts (ready to bake), bread, leftover flour from milling (for muffins, cakes, cookies, etc.), leftover flaked cereals (for cereal, breads, muffins, cookies, etc.).

These pantries are filled with delicious possibilities. There are no chemical additives, coloring, or artificial flavors in whole foods.

Learn to Prepare and Present Life-Giving Foods Which Appeal to Both the Eye and the Palate

We must accomplish three goals when we serve a breakfast, lunch or dinner, light supper, high tea, or snack.

1) To give our bodies the foods we require to build healthy cells;

2) To select cooking techniques which will not produce cancer-causing agents;

3) To present foods which are a delight to the senses—in an atmosphere which brings joy to the hearts—of those we serve.

Building Healthy Cells

Life begins and ends at the cellular level. We need to understand the connection between the Lord's provision of food and the effects these foods have on the cells in our bodies. We have discussed the foods which meet our need for macronutrients: carbohydrates, proteins, and lipids. We know that eating grains, beans, fruit, vegetables, and essential fatty acids are the healthiest way in which any of us can consume the macronutrients we need. We have also mentioned three micronutrients: vitamins, minerals, and amino acids. Likewise, consuming grains, legumes, fruits, vegetables, and essential fatty acids enable us to meet the requirements our bodies have for these micronutrients. We have not, however, discussed in sufficient detail our need for a fourth type of micronutrient—enzymes.

The human body has more than three thousand enzymes, and without them we could not function. Life would cease. Where do they come from? All uncooked food. Whenever we heat food much above the human body temperature, the enzymes in that food are no longer able to perform their function. Each type of enzyme fulfills a specific function. While nutritionists and dietitians often remind us that nutrients abound in cooked food—and they do—they often fail to mention that cooking food totally destroys the enzyme activity. This is a very great problem because we need enzymes in order to digest our food. Our bodies need enzymes in order to break protein into amino acids. Without them, our bodies could not store sugar in the liver, turn fat into fatty tissue, turn phosphorous into bone, or attach iron to red blood cells.[65]

Therefore, in planning our meals we need to include raw vegetables and raw fruits. Any breakfast, lunch, dinner, or snack can feature a large bowl or plate filled with diced or shredded raw vegetables, served alone or with grains or legumes. We prefer to eat raw vegetables for the first two meals of the day and then eat cooked food, vegetables, grains, and, perhaps, beans for supper. My husband eats a raw fruit lunch, followed by a large salad with grains in the middle to late afternoon.

> Enzymes are the catalyst in the chemical reactions that continually take place in our bodies. They cause these reactions to happen, and they regulate the speed at which they occur. Although enzymes are intimately involved in the chemistry of life, they themselves remain unchanged. They facilitate reactions but are not reacted on themselves.[66]

Fresh fruit and vegetables, served raw; freshly extracted raw vegetable and fruit juice; and certain whole foods concentrates all provide ample live enzymes. They are not just good foods which make us a bit healthier, they are foods which prevent and cure disease and sustain life. Sometimes people simply cannot tolerate raw fruits or vegetables; freshly extracted juice or whole foods concentrates are the answer. In Step Four, we discuss the advantages of whole foods concentrates more thoroughly.

Healthful Cooking Techniques

Those who decide to continue eating meat regularly or occasionally need to know how meat should be cooked. According to Richard H. Adamson, Ph.D., at the National Cancer Institute, stewing, boiling, and poaching are the methods which do not produce cancer-causing agents. These cancer-causing agents are called heterocyclic aromatic amines (HAAs).

Frying, grilling, broiling, and barbecuing produce large numbers of these agents. Oven roasting and baking produces moderate amounts of HAAs. In the cells, these HAAs damage the DNA, thus preparing the body for cancer. HAAs have been fed to numerous animals in the laboratories causing a wide variety of cancer.[67]

Turkeys and chickens are easily steamed whole in large pots on top of the stove (use pots with tightly fitting lids). Poaching is a traditional method of preparing fish and works quite well. Beef and lamb, as well as poultry, can be diced and cooked in pots of soup or stew. It makes little sense to buy meat which is free of hormones and pesticides and then produce cancer-causing agents during the cooking process.

Food Which Delights the Senses and an Atmosphere Which Brings Joy to the Heart

This topic warrants a full day seminar or a full year of weekly cooking classes. There are many, many books on the subject of preparing healthful foods. But, we don't need a lot of information in order to get started. We begin with complex carbohydrates. Steamed rice, spelt, or barley are foods which sustain us and make a wonderful foundation for any meal. Then we need to think of serving a variety of colors, flavors, and textures. Both cooked and raw vegetables can be used to make an interesting and delicious dinner. Here is a simple example (and no recipes are necessary):

Grain (beige or brown in color)

Sweet potato or squash (orange or yellow in color)

Greens of some sort (dark green)

Mixed raw cruciferous vegetables:

Cauliflower (white)

Cabbage (light green or purple)

Radishes (red and white)

Broccoli (dark green)

Beans (red, white, or beige)

The grain is chewy. The sweet potatoes are soft and sweet. The raw vegetables are crunchy. The tastes range from sweet to sour. Garlic, onions, and herbs add variety.

Think about the simplicity in food preparation. The grains and beans are prepared ahead of time. We needn't stand over a hot stove. Sweet potatoes and squash are rinsed, poked with a knife, and baked in the oven. Again, we don't stand over a stove. Greens are washed, cut, steamed, and seasoned with herbs, garlic, and onions. The most time consuming part of this particular meal is shredding and dicing the vegetables for the large bowl of mixed raw vegetables, which we serve seasoned with extra virgin olive oil and raw apple cider vinegar.

For hundreds of recipe ideas, you may want to collect cookbooks which have been written by people who follow vegan diets (no meat, poultry, fish, eggs, or dairy). Recipes which contain meat and meat products abound; the others are harder to find and very useful. Here are the vegetarian authors which I recommend most highly.

• *Eat for Strength* (has an Oil Free Edition) by Agatha Thrash, M.D.

• *Of These Ye May Freely Eat* by JoAnn Rachor

• *The Country Life Vegetarian Cookbook* (from the kitchens of Country Life Vegetarian Restaurants) edited by Diana J. Fleming

• *Recipes from the Weimar Kitchen* (Weimer Institute)

• *Cooking with Natural Foods (Books I & II)* by Muriel Beltz

(For more information see "Resource Guide.")

Finally, if we purpose to delight in the tasks at hand, we will bring joy to those we serve. What could we be doing that is more important than taking care of those over whom God has given us charge, than nurturing those we love and support, than strengthening our own bodies that we may serve Him?

If we learn to take care of ourselves and our families as the Lord leads us, we can depend upon Him to provide us with the strength, compassion, and love to do the work at hand. When the Lord gives us the grace to walk in any truth, He also allows a time of trial, a time to face temptation. Encountering rejection while seeking to do what is right is not an odd thing, but, rather, the usual thing (1 Pet. 8:12). And, through our obedience to God, in the difficult times and in the pleasant times, we learn to walk in peace and joy. Our husbands, children, friends, relatives, and strangers will respond to His Spirit according to His will. We can rest in that. Our responsibility is to put on the whole armor of God in order that we "may be able to stand firm against the schemes of the devil" (Eph. 6:11).

Those we love who have been eating toaster pastries for breakfast; hamburgers, white buns, and french fries for lunch; and precooked, packaged meals for dinner may be determined to continue making poor food choices in spite of all warnings and exhortations. Or, they may suddenly decide to leap into a healthy lifestyle in a single bound. Jesus is Lord over all. He is patient and merciful. We need not become desperate because our spouses or children or parents or parents-in-law or friends haven't had the same revelation that we have had. Many people only become interested in changing their dietary regimes after they have experienced health problems. No matter how we come to the point where we recognize our problems and seek His help in solving them, we must acknowledge that God is the one who brings us to the point of confession and repentance. As we give God the glory for the needs He meets in our own lives, others will see His hand of mercy, and by His grace they will reach out for help as well. If we condemn others and judge them for their weaknesses, then we fail to see our own greater weaknesses: "And why do you look at the speck that is in your brother's eye, but do not notice the log that is in your own" (Luke 6:41)?

The mystery of godliness is that the work is His: "For we are His workmanship, created in Christ Jesus for good works, which God prepared beforehand, that we should walk in them" (Eph. 2:10).

When we walk in wisdom—in any area—our lives can be a lifeline. But, without eyes to see, those in need cannot reach out to be rescued. Only the Lord can prepare the hearts of His people. He is calling us to love one another and to pray for one another that we may be healed. He hears, and He answers prayer. And, as we pray, God will reveal to us our own great sin and need. The message to us from 1 Peter is to keep fervent in love:

> Above all, keep fervent in love for one another, because love covers a multitude of sins. Be hospitable to one another without complaint. As each one has received a special gift, employ it in serving

one another, as good stewards of the manifold grace of God.

Whoever speaks, let him speak, as it were, the utterances of God; whoever serves, let him do so as by the strength which God supplies; so that in all things God may be glorified through Jesus Christ, to whom belongs the glory and dominion forever and ever. (1 Pet. 4:8–11)

Step Three

Make Time for Life-Saving, Life-Enhancing Activities

Preparation:

Discover the compelling reasons for consuming products made from freshly milled flour.

Examine the nutritional benefits of dehydrated foods over frozen and canned foods.

Consider the value of having a reliable supply of pure and powerful food–365 days a year–growing right in your own kitchen.

Milling and Baking:
The Delicious Way to Build Health

Once we realize that products made from commercially milled flour are devoid of essential fiber and nutrients, we are wise to examine the alternatives: 1) we can stop eating bread, muffins, cakes, cookies, rolls, pancakes, waffles, and pasta which have been made from commercially milled flour; 2) we can try to find a business willing to mill flour for us and to make the baked goods we need; 3) we can try to find an individual who is willing to both mill the flour and make the products which we desire; 4) we can purchase a home flour mill and a breadmaker-mixer and learn to make the wonderful products which we want and need; or 5) we can continue eating products made from commercially milled flour even though such products destroy our health. Many people decide to continue eating baked goods which are devitalized and lacking in fiber and nutrients—simply because they are tasty and

141

convenient. A few people are able to find a "health bakery" which operates as both a mill and bakery and produces wholesome products. But, the most satisfying, liberating, life-changing and life-enhancing solution of all is to buy a home flour mill and breadmaker-mixer and learn to use them.

By milling beans and grains, we produce flour products which are rich in essential nutrients, insoluble fiber, and soluble fiber. Baked goods, as well as cereals and pasta products, made from freshly milled flour are not only life-giving, they are far more delicious than any products made from commercially milled flour.

Commercial millers remove the bran, the protective layer around each kernel of grain. The absence of bran in our diets is a major cause of degenerative disease. A nutritional clinic in England gave patients apples, carrots, cabbage, and wheat bran in order to compare the effectiveness of various types of vegetable fibers as a source of bulk in the diet. They concluded that although vegetables were useful, nothing came close to the effectiveness of wheat bran. I have personally advised hundreds of people to begin eating bread made from freshly milled flour. The results are always the same: the weight of the stool increases; the stool is softer; and the transit time decreases. The bran we get in the freshly milled flour not only prevents constipation but prevents bowel and colon cancer as well. Bran is an insoluble fiber which remains unchanged in the digestive process and removes fat from the walls of the colon and clears our bodies of unwanted metals and toxins. In the wheat kernel, these outer layers (removed in the commercial refining process) contain 86 percent of the niacin in the whole kernel of wheat, 73 percent of the pyridoxine, 50 percent of the pantothenic acid, 42 percent of the riboflavin, 33 percent of the thiamine, and 19 percent of the protein. These nutrients—and all of the vital fiber—are removed in the refining process which turns whole grain flour into white flour and brown rice into white rice. Dr. Denis P. Burkitt, the famous British surgeon who is responsible for alerting the medical community to the critical need for fiber, observed that degenerative diseases occur in a particular order in cultures which westernize their diets. The diseases emerge gradually, in steps of progressive degeneration.[1] As societies westernize, they first begin to experience incidences of appendicitis, then hemorrhoids and varicose veins; colon polyps, colon cancer, hiatal hernia, and diverticular disease follow.

According to Dr. Denis Burkitt, the average American adult passes eighty to one hundred and twenty grams of stool a day. The average person in Africa, India, the Pacific Islands, and other countries passes three hundred to five hundred grams of stool a day. These high stool weights and low transit times are associated with low occurrence of Western diseases. Dr. Neal Barnard observes in his recent work, that the diet of the average Westerner supplies only about ten to twenty grams of fiber.[2] People whose diet centers around meat, fried potatoes, soft drinks, sugar, and products made from refined flour often consume even less fiber than the national average.

Researchers at the University of Lund, in Sweden, have found that fiber in the diet can absorb known compounds (quinolines) which are very potent carcinogens (cancer-causing agents). The fiber from wheat and other grains has the capacity to leach out up to 20 percent of these compounds. Therefore, the presence of fiber is important for three reasons: first, it increases and softens the bulk of the stool by absorbing water; second, it decreases the transit time of the stool in the intestinal tract; and third, it absorbs cancer-causing compounds which may be in the diet. This means that the more fiber we consume, the more we reduce the length of time that cancer-causing agents will actually be able to remain in contact with the intestinal lining. The outer layer of every grain provides nutritionally rich, insoluble fiber which we now know is a vital component of good health.

After the bran with its essential nutrients and fiber are removed from the wheat berry, the commercial millers remove the middling. This nutritious second layer is then sold to the farmers as an excellent source of feed for animals. Finally, they remove the wheat germ, the most nutritious part of the wheat berry. The wheat germ oil is one of the richest sources of vitamin E, vitamin B-complex, and high-quality protein. Ninety percent of the nutritional value of the wheat berry is in the wheat germ. However, wheat germ must be removed from all commercial flour—even so-called whole wheat flour—because wheat germ oil has a short shelf life and becomes rancid very quickly. Rancid oil is both unpleasant tasting and carcinogenic. By consuming the flour made from freshly milled wheat berries we get the benefit of twenty-five vitamins, minerals, and proteins, as well as the important benefit of the bran.

We can improve the nutritional value of all our baked goods by using 20 percent bean flour. I prefer to mill the mild-tasting white beans or garbanzo beans for baking purposes. The soluble fiber in the bean flour has an important benefit: it actually breaks down to form a gel in the small intestines, retarding the absorption of glucose. This is highly significant for those who suffer from diabetes or hypoglycemia; it protects them from the rapid breakdown of carbohydrates. It is the rapid breakdown of carbohydrates which makes it quite difficult to manage those diseases. A recipe using a variety of grains and beans is found in Ezekiel 4:9 and is often referred to as Ezekiel Bread:

> Take thou also unto thee wheat, and barley, and beans, and lentils, and millet, and fitches, and put them into one vessel, and make thee bread thereof . . .

Beans help lower blood pressure, reduce "bad" cholesterol, and, often, prevent and cure both constipation and hemorrhoids. Protease inhibitors, a basic component of beans, are effective in blocking certain cancers including colon and breast cancer. These protease inhibitors may be more effective in preventing cancer than they are in curing it: they are effective in stopping out-of-control cell division before such division progresses to cancer.

Although nearly everyone likes the goodness of "real bread" made from freshly milled wheat berries, most people are also glad to discover the many health benefits and delightful flavors found in many other grains and in bean flours. Instead of consuming devitalized products made from commercially milled flour—products which actually cause disease—we can produce a wide variety of delicious, life-saving baked goods made from grains and beans which we mill right in our own homes. The appliances which are now available make milling and baking simple and gratifying tasks. These machines do the work of many servants. Some of the busiest and most productive people we know take time to mill their own flour for breads and pasta and flake their own grain for cereal. Taking time to do tasks which enable us to provide life-giving food for our families is an act of love that multiplies our time. How? When we are stronger and healthier, we are able to take full advantage of the hours which God has given us. We also learn to enjoy doing those very tasks which are life-giving. By His grace, less important occupations eventually lose their hold on us.

How to Find a Mill and a Breadmaker-Mixer

As I mentioned in Part One, after my husband and I discovered the advantages of freshly milled flour, we began searching for the ideal home flour mill. Like most people, we thought "stone mills" represented a back-to-the-best, old-methods-are-better approach. Then, after looking at a number of machines and manufacturers, we discovered Magic Mill, a small mill and mixer company in Salt Lake City, Utah. As we began doing marketing for them, we evaluated all of the home flour mills, breadmaker-mixers and dehydrators on the market. Our findings concerning the range of products available are beyond the scope of this work. However, as a result of our work, many of our friends, acquaintances, and family members felt compelled to begin milling and baking. And, in order to accomplish those tasks, they chose to purchase the same machines which we use. Our advice to every consumer who is shopping for a home flour mill and a breadmaker-mixer is this: 1) contact the manufacturers of the appliances you are considering and request the names of dealers who will show you each machine in operation; 2) if the manufacturers cannot give you the names of dealers in your area, obtain video tapes showing the machines in operation; 3) be certain that there are money-back guarantees on the machines; and 4) be certain that the machines are under warranty.

Thom Leonard is a writer, farmer, and a baker. His book, *The Bread Book*, is a delightful work which offers tips on choosing a home flour mill, growing grains and harvesting them, and building a wood-fired brick oven. And, although I have chosen to do activities which leave me no time to do many of the tasks which Mr. Leonard does, I find many of his goals and accomplishments pleasant to consider. He does not discuss breadmaker-mixers in his book because he believes it is best to knead the dough by hand. Like many of the people that I counsel, I need machines which will accelerate the time in which these baking tasks can be done. I recommend Mr. Leonard's book to many of my friends who think that they cannot possibly face one more challenge in their busy lives. Compared to growing grain, kneading dough by hand, and cooking in a wood-fired brick oven, it is incredibly easy to begin milling and baking according to the methods which I suggest. Mr. Leonard offers his evaluation of various mills ranging in price from over two hundred dollars to over eight hundred dollars. He prefers stone mills over micronizing mills but offers a very useful discussion concerning the choices between the two micronizing mills on the market. The price of the Magic Mill Home Flour Mill has changed significantly since he wrote *The Bread Book*. Since Magic Mill now operates as a wholesale buying club, consumers who pay a small fee (under twenty dollars) can buy their products and appliances at wholesale prices.

Nutriflex has managed well with this arrangement because they are able to sell directly to the consumer at the same prices they once charged their dealers. Furthermore, many of the customers who at the outset were only interested in buying machines at wholesale prices have now become acquainted with a wide range of products which are offered by this health and fitness company. Not only can they purchase dough enhancer and pro-wheat gluten for baking, they can buy an organic all-purpose kitchen cleaner which is totally botanical and a wide range of other health-oriented products as well. Nutriflex is able to offer the machines at such low prices because the people who buy the machines spread the word even more effectively than dealers once did: dealers made a profit on each machine; members of a network marketing company simply offer people the opportunity to buy wholesale. Network marketing works when people get a legitimately good, or even great, value. However, there is no obligation to make any purchase from Nutriflex after buying the machines at wholesale. Anyone who wants to pay the membership fee, purchase the appliances wholesale, and never order from the company again is free to do so. All of the products can be ordered by calling a toll-free number.

Here are some of Thom Leonard's remarks concerning micronizing mills:

> The Magic Mill outperformed the Kitchen Mill (K-Tech) on several counts. It is almost three times as fast, created less dust (the Kitchen Mill blew flour past its filter), was more willing to accept large kernels of corn, created less of a temperature rise, and held more grain in the hopper and more flour in the catch pan. Both produced extremely fine flour on the next-to-finest setting. The Lexan plastic mill body on the Kitchen Mill was cracked upon arrival, but it performed well regardless. While the Magic Mill has a stainless steel flour pan that locks in place with spring-loaded steel balls, the Kitchen Mill has a smoke-tint Lexan pan that is held in place

with molded clips on the side of the mill housing.
I wouldn't trust these to continued use, especially
considering the condition the mill arrived in. Plastic is not the most resilient and durable material
under stress or tension.[3]

Thom Leonard does not care for noise and space age
technology. What mill did he choose?

> With its wooden housing and natural stones, the
> Kootenay A-130 comes closest to satisfying my aes-
> thetic needs. It also grinds satisfactory flour from
> all grains except the hardest flint corn, and even
> that was usable. It is simple to operate, fast, and
> relatively cool-grinding. With a retail price of around
> $650 (depending on the exchange rate) it is not
> inexpensive, but there are more expensive mills.[4]

But, what is his recommendation for those of us who
do not mind the noise a mill might make (we use ear
plugs) and who do find the speed at which flour is milled
and the cost of the mill itself to be crucial considerations?

> While the noise and basic construction are enough
> to make me shy away from the two micronizers,
> they do grind fine flour quickly. If I had to choose
> between the two I'd take the Magic Mill III Plus.[5]

In order to gain insight concerning all of the possibilities regarding the purchase of a home flour mill, consumers need to read reviews by competent bakers who live in
contrasting cultures and have different sets of priorities.
Thom Leonard's book is small, easy to read, and available
through interlibrary loan. In the *Eating Better Program Guide*
which I wrote for Magic Mill Nutriflex, I share these conclusions about the various types of home flour mills available:

> Historically, milling has been accomplished by crush-
> ing and grinding the grains between large heavy
> stones. Today's home mills operate by one of three
> means: abrasive grit wheels, cone-and burr mecha-
> nism or Micro-Milling™ heads. "Stone" mills actu-

ally employ a pair of abrasive grit wheels, similar to what is used in a machine shop for grinding or sharpening metal objects. They are effective, (although they are slow); tend to leave grit on the flour; and sometimes glaze over and require cleaning. Cone-and-burr mills use a nested cone-shaped mechanism, usually made of stainless steel. The inner cone has a sharply ribbed texture and rotates, grinding the wheat against the smooth fixed outer cone. The process is slow, and the flour produced is somewhat coarser than what is produced by other methods. In contrast, Micro-Milling™ heads operate by a unique high-speed impact principle, rather than by grinding. When a grain or bean enters the milling chamber, surgical stainless steel teeth, rotating at up to 28,000 rpm collide with it, exploding it and then instantly refining the particles into a beautifully fine flour. The process is extremely fast, and leaves no foreign particles in the flour. Because there is very little friction, a very high rate of flour production can be achieved, without significantly elevating the temperature of the flour. This is the technology used in the Magic Mill Plus Home Flour Mill.[6]

After Gary and I discovered the many features offered in the home flour mills available, we had no difficulty deciding what features were most important to us. We wanted a lightweight, compact, reasonably priced piece of equipment with an incredibly good warranty (five years). We definitely wanted self-cleaning surgical steel milling heads and, perhaps most important, a high-speed operation (1.2 pounds of commercial grade flour per minute). We needed to see the mill in operation, feel and smell the flour, and taste the products made from the flour just after they came out of the oven. Anyone who is ready to purchase equipment should attempt to see just such a demonstration.

Buying a breadmaker-mixer is a truly simple matter for the educated consumer. Many people think that the Kitchen

Aid is the finest kitchen machine on the market world-wide. It is a good mixer which is widely advertised in the United States. However, Electrolux of Sweden manufactures the DLX Breadmaker-mixer, a complete kitchen center, which has been on the European market for over fifty years. The machine kneads up to fifteen pounds of dough without giving the motor the slightest strain (or without walking on the counter). The extra-capacity, seamless stainless steel bowl sets the standard for quality, durability, hygiene, and capacity. Two qualities assure hygiene: the stainless steel bowl can withstand extreme temperatures, and there are no seams or shafts in the bowl where bacteria can collect. The absence of a center cone makes mixing convenient and cleaning easy.

With the help of this heavy-duty machine, available wholesale through Nutriflex, anyone can prepare a wide variety of whole grain products quickly and easily. The Flake Mill attachment turns oat groats, wheat berries, barley, spelt, and other grains into flakes which can be used in cereals, breakfast bars, cookies, muffins, and other baked goods. The Pasta Maker creates real excitement; the favorite food of so many people becomes a feast filled with fiber and nutrients! Our children would like a side dish of pasta with every meal, and, with the Pasta Maker, we are happy to accommodate them.

Recently, I spoke to a professional baker who owns the DLX Breadmaker-mixer. She agreed that there is no close second to this machine. At nearly the same price, other machines which are currently on the market cannot begin to perform the same tasks. I asked my baker-friend about the larger, commercial machines which could produce more dough. She said that in order to buy a machine which could perform as well as the DLX, she would have to buy a commercial breadmaker-mixer at a cost of several thousand dollars. Instead, for her small operation, she is going to purchase a second DLX. The DLX is currently available direct to the consumer for just over four hundred dollars.

The Advantages of Advanced Food Dehydration

Dehydration, as a means of preserving fruits and vegetables, is superior to both freezing and canning. The FDA confirms that 20 to 30 percent of the nutrients are retained in canned foods; 40 to 60 percent are retained in frozen foods; and 95 to 97 percent are retained in dehydrated foods.

Not only is dehydration the most nutritious method, it is the quickest and easiest method. After the food is dehydrated, storage is not a problem: one hundred tomatoes, dried and powdered, fit into a quart jar. The powder can be reconstituted as we need it for pasta sauce, pizza sauce, and other tomato products.

A wide variety of foods can be processed: fruits, vegetables, herbs, meat, poultry, and fish. All of these foods can be dried as chips or powdered for use as soup stock or seasoning. Dehydration assures us of a pantry which is never empty, but is filled with foods which are free from food additives and preservatives. While we are sleeping, the machine dries the foods efficiently and safely.

Dehydrated snacks are ideal substitutes for sugar-filled treats and high-fat corn and potato chips. Fruit leathers are a favorite among children and adults. Fruit chips are delicious with homemade museli or trail mix. (Homemade museli: dehydrated apple chips, or other fruit chips, crushed walnuts, freshly flaked oat groats, juice of half a lemon, barley malt syrup.) Vegetable chips are both colorful and pleasing when flavored with herbal seasonings. Their crunchy texture satisfies the craving for chips which many people experience as they make the change from a high-fat, low-fiber diet to a high-fiber, low-fat diet. Experiencing a variety of tastes and textures helps make the transition easier.

It is essential that we use a dehydrator which is completely reliable. Many inefficient dehydrators are on the market, and the problems they cause are serious ones. According to experts at University Extension Services, a dehydrator must reach 138 degrees to 145 degrees in order to prevent contamination. If food is not dried properly, it actually presents a health risk. Some people want to use machines which permit a lower drying temperature. This, they insist, will not kill the live enzymes in the dehydrated food. After talking to numerous food scientists regarding this matter, I am convinced that we need to go ahead and kill the enzymes rather than risk the threat of disease. One expert at a University Extension Service told me that dehydrating food at an improper temperature could allow contamination which could result in death. The advanced dehydrator which we use has 100 percent solid state circuitry and precisely controls the drying temperature to plus or minus five degrees of optimum. It adjusts the temperature 120 times per second with total accuracy. It dries food uniformly and consistently at a very low cost. Because the machine uses forced air instead of convection, it allows a shorter drying time and prevents food spoilage.

Raw fruits and vegetables, as well as sprouts and whole foods concentrates, are the best source of live enzymes. We do not consider dehydrated foods a source of live enzymes. Dehydrating our foods offers convenience and pleasure; safety is a major consideration. Dehydrated foods are highly nutritious "fast foods" for those times when we are on the go; they are also ideal foods for the pantry because they offer instant meals.

Drying times for vegetables range from two to ten hours; for fruits, four to fourteen hours. We simply place the products onto the dehydration trays and let the machine do the work. We can store the products in plastic storage bags or glass jars.

Power Foods from Your Own Kitchen

Homegrown sprouts—"power foods"

Sprouts are among the most perfect foods we can consume. Sprouting is a process which increases the nutritional value of seeds, grains, and legumes. When these foods are sprouted, their food value increases 30 to 600 percent. If the sprouts are allowed to turn green, they are a rich source of chlorophyll and other important nutrients. Sprouting also adds enzymes which change starches to sugars and proteins to amino acids. Vitamin C increases up to 600 percent in many instances. Certainly, the nutrients in sprouts are more easily assimilated than those contained in isolated nutrients.

Obtaining Seeds

The purpose of sprouting is to obtain a totally reliable, highly nutritious, pure food supply 365 days out of the year. It is therefore unwise to use anything except certified organic seeds. OCIA, OGBA, FVO, and others are independent third parties who verify that the seed has been grown according to certain standards. If the local health food store cannot offer all of the help that you need, then contact one of the grain specialists listed in Step Two. He offers booklets about sprouting and useful supplies.

Sprouts grow rapidly and easily. In the right combination, they give us all that we need for health. All sprouts contain vitamins, minerals, trace minerals, enzymes, and fiber. With sprouts, we can grow organic vegetables in our own home every day of the year.

Popular seeds to sprout are alfalfa, mung beans, aduki, soy, garbanzo, kidney, pinto, lima and fava beans, fenugreek, lentils, peas, wheat, buckwheat, oats, rye, and corn.

Sprouting can be done in jars, trays, sacks, or a colander. If we start small quantities of sprouts every few days, then we always have a fresh supply of sprouts. The nutrients in sprouts begin to deteriorate after two to three days. They need to be consumed as soon as they reach their prime. Also, we eat the entire sprout—seed, root, leaf, and skin. All of us, even small children, can prepare sprouts. We have only to place value on acquiring habits which are life-giving. We can begin by growing a delightful tray of sprouts ourselves and, then, by serving them.

Acquiring Life-Giving Skills

As we consider each of these simple, life-enhancing, life-saving tasks, we need to evaluate the quality of our lives and the significance that lies in simple things. What are the delights that a family shares by milling flour and baking bread together? How do we profit by watering a jar of seeds and watching them explode with essential nutrients? What is the importance of making a provision for the future by filling our pantries with fruits and vegetables which will meet our nutritional needs and bring pleasure as well. May God make us careful, sensitive people who regard nurturing and sustaining one another as the essential business of our lives. May we thank Him for giving us the energy to serve each other and the grace to see His love in the tasks at hand.

Prevent or Cure Degenerative Disease

Preparation:

Recognize the environmental dangers which exist in our country and around the world.

Evaluate the reasons for drinking safe water.

Understand the ways in which foods heal the body.

Accept the overwhelming evidence that the dehydrated green juice of young barley leaves is one of the richest sources of all nutrients available in any form anywhere.

Understand the essentials of oral hygiene in order to prevent gum disease, loss of teeth, and halitosis.

Seek medical treatment from those who recognize Jesus Christ as our Healer and Great Physician, who understand the healing power of food, and who give hope to those the world calls "hopeless" through nutritional therapy.

Water

Although it has been widely publicized that the public water treatment facilities in our country are not equipped to cope with the many deadly chemicals, radioactive wastes, and other contaminants in our water, people still drink the water which is provided by our cities without filtering, distilling, or treating it in any way. The pollutants in the water supply itself are only part of the problem; the city and household plumbing in most communities also pose a significant threat to the purity of the water. Consuming pure water is essential to achieving optimal health. We need to recognize the fact that this country has a major water contamination problem and that the problem is getting worse. We need to take action to protect ourselves and our families. And we have a responsibility to share the information with others who are in danger by drinking contaminated water.

Even so-called approved water (approved under the Environmental Protection Agency standards) may contain numerous poisons—lead, arsenic, mercury, and radioactive particles. Cancer-causing chemicals such as trichloroethylene (TCE), chloroform (from chlorine), DBCP (a farm and garden pesticide), and alachor (the nation's most widely used pesticide) are showing up all across the country. Lists of contaminants literally fill books. The EPA has also announced that the water supply in many older homes contains dangerous levels of lead and copper due to the age of the plumbing. According to the United States Geological Survey, there are contaminated water supplies both above and below ground in every state. Our public water treatment facilities are not equipped to detect or evaluate problems of this magnitude, and they certainly aren't prepared to eliminate these problems.

The "approved" solutions to the problems with our drinking water pose significant health risks as well. First is the problem of chlorine. Many experts believe that chlorine and its byproducts can cause cancer, heart disease, kidney stones, diabetes, and other diseases. Some treatment facilities add fluoride to the water. Drinking water treated with fluoride can interfere with thyroid function and create a number of other health problems. But, the threat of degenerative disease seems remote to many people. Unless the cause of illness and death can be traced directly to the water, many choose to look the other way. The direct threat is now here—cryptosporidium.

In 1993, an estimated four hundred thousand people fell ill as a result of the presence of this parasite in the drinking water in Milwaukee; forty-one thousand were treated for abdominal cramps and diarrhea; four thousand were hospitalized; and 104 people died in the epidemic. It was the single largest medical disaster in Milwaukee's history. *USA Today* published these observations in July 1994:

> Last year's water crisis in Milwaukee, in which more than 100 people died and thousands became ill, was merely a wake-up call, says Carolyn Hartmann of the U.S. Public Interest Research Group. It is completely hypocritical for Congress to claim they are concerned about health-care reform and then turn around and vote for a bill that threatens our drinking water.

> U.S. health officials estimate 900,000 people each year become ill—and possibly 900 die—from water-borne disease. The General Accounting Office estimates 66% of Safe Drinking Water Act violations aren't reported.[1]

Cryptosporidium is a pathogenic protozoan. The eggs of this parasite have a rugged shell which makes chlorine ineffective in killing them. After the eggs have hatched inside the intestinal tract, they feed off the nutrients inside the cells of the small intestine. If we boil our water in order to kill the cryptosporidium, we end up with a pan filled with lead, copper, sodium, nitrates, and other contaminants. The best solution is to distill our water at home and to buy distilled water when we are away from home. The next best solution is water filtered by reverse osmosis.

The Natural Resources Defense Council issued a study in March of 1994 which stated that more than 90 percent of the major water utilities have failed to install post-World War I technologies to remove the contaminants from the water supply. According to the *Orlando Sentinel,* our water is not up to standards:

> The report said most, major water suppliers have done little to prevent contamination of watersheds or groundwater, have not installed modern equipment to fight chemical contamination and many do

not use basic technologies to remove microbiologi-
cal contamination from their water.

Chlorine is widely used to disinfect water, but the
report said it is not being treated against cancer-
linked byproducts formed by a reaction with organic materials.[2]

According to an article in *USA Today*, the study by the
Natural Resources Defense Council indicates that the most
pervasive contaminants are coliform bacteria, cancer-causing trihalomethanes, radioactive elements, and lead.[3]

We purchased an expensive reverse osmosis system
several years ago; but after reviewing all of the distillation
and reverse osmosis systems currently available, we think
that the Waterwise 7000 with its precarbon and postcarbon
filters is the best home system today. For information comparing the various methods of water purification see the
Resource Guide.

Pure water is essential for optimal health. Finding a
reliable source of pure water is a wise endeavor. Drinking
tap water, anywhere in America, at anytime, is certainly a
hazard which informed people ought to avoid.

A Diet Restricted to "Power Foods"

A year after my own health had been restored, I began
studying the diets which physicians find most useful in
curing specific degenerative diseases: Dr. Dean Ornish's
diet used in connection with his program for reversing
heart disease; Dr. Collin H. Dong's diet for curing arthritis; the Exclusion Diet for eliminating food intolerances
developed by Dr. John Hunter and Dr. Virginia Alun Jones;
and Dr. William G. Crook's dietary guidelines for those
who suffer with candida. The physicians who worked with
food intolerances and candida provided me with real insight into the connection between the symptoms that I had
suffered and the foods that I had been eating. However, I
noticed that on each physician's recommended list were
devitalized foods or foods high in fat: e.g., sugar, white
flour, meat or sunflower oil, soy oil and safflower oil,

margarine, nuts, or white rice. Although some of the patients "tolerate" some of these foods and still get relief from the specific diseases these physicians are treating, devitalized foods don't build optimal health. It is worth our while to examine the "exclusions" and "inclusions" on each of these lists because there are a group of foods which seem to offend no one and another group of foods which offend many people. By sorting out that information I saved thousands of dollars, precious time, and regained my health. There are a group of "power foods" which provide a place for everyone to begin, no matter what their symptoms. We may be examined by the most brilliant diagnostician in the world and lose our lives. The medical profession has gained amazing expertise in diagnosing conditions, but the death toll rises. And yet, people can be and are being cured without ever discovering what is wrong with them—simply by consuming foods that heal! We need to remember that each of these physicians has a verifiable record of success in treating a specific disease with a specific diet.

Dr. Dean Ornish's Diet for Reversing Heart Disease

Dr. Dean Ornish's diet for reversing heart disease excludes all animal products except nonfat milk, nonfat yogurt, and egg whites. He excludes all meat, poultry, fish, egg yolks, and dairy (other than the nonfat dairy mentioned). He excludes one vegetable, olives, which are high in fat, and one fruit, avocados, which are also high in fat. He excludes all other vegetarian food which is high in fat: nuts, seeds, all oils, chocolate, all cocoa products, and coconut. He excludes caffeine, all other stimulants, and monosodium glutamate. He does not restrict calories in his program for reversing heart disease.[4]

Dr. Ornish recommends that anyone with a cholesterol level over 150 follow the Reversal Diet. The diet includes all grains and beans. It includes all vegetables and fruits other than the high-fat ones mentioned. With this regime one consumes less than 10 percent of calories from fat and very little of it is saturated. Dr. Ornish doesn't encourage alcohol consumption, but his program allows less than two ounces a day for those who consume alcohol. He allows moderate use of salt and sugar. The recipes he recommends call for a variety of flours, and there is no mention of the value in using freshly milled flour. Since there is no emphasis on intact grains as opposed to devitalized flour, it does not feature optimal nutrition. The strength of the diet, which he developed as part of a program which reverses heart disease without drugs and surgery, is that it is low in fat. He says that patients are able to get omega-3 fatty acids from "whole grains, beans, seaweed and soybean products."[5]

As we mentioned in Step Two, scientists who study the benefits of omega-3 fatty acids tell us that the best sources are seeds, plants from cold climates, green leafy vegetables, and oils extracted from cold-water fish like mackerel, salmon, tuna, or cod. Flaxseed oil is the best source available. Unless we understand our need for omega-3 fatty acid and recognize the sources which will satisfy that need, it is unlikely that we will consume the essential fatty acids which we need for optimal health. Certainly, those who consume a generous amount of green, leafy vegetables daily will get enough essential (omega-3) fatty acids, but few people eat an adequate supply of green leafy vegetables on a regular basis. Dr. Ornish recommends several foods in his program which cannot be considered foods for building optimal health: nonfat dairy, sugar, and refined flour products. Dr. Ornish's program, which includes the diet we have just mentioned, is the only system scientifically proven to reverse heart disease without drugs or surgery.

Dr. Collin Dong's Diet for Curing Arthritis

Dr. Dong's diet for curing arthritis excludes all red meat, poultry, and egg yolks (he allows egg whites); all fruit, including tomatoes; and all dairy, including milk, cheese, and yogurt; vinegar, pepper, monosodium glutamate; alcohol; soft drinks; all additives, preservatives, and chemicals. Dr. Dong's diet includes a wide variety of foods, a great many of which are not health-building. Included are all seafoods; all vegetables, including avocado; vegetable oils, particular safflower and corn; margarines free of milk solids, such as Mazola; egg whites; honey; nuts, sunflower seeds, soybean products; rice of all kinds—brown, white, wild; bread which has no ingredients which are listed on the exclusion list; tea and coffee; plain soda water; parsley, onions, garlic, bay leaf, salt; any kind of flour; and sugar.[6]

Dr. Dong recommends a number of foods for arthritics which cannot be considered foods which help us achieve optimal health: all seafoods (many of these are filled with cholesterol and most are filled with contaminants); egg whites; margarine (contains transfatty acids); safflower and corn oils (extra virgin olive oil and flaxseed oil are the good choices); devitalized white rice and white flour; sugar; and tea and coffee. Dr. Dong's diet has been used effectively in treating arthritis.

Doctors John Hunter and Virginia Alun Jones's Exclusion Diet

The Exclusion Diet for Food Intolerance, advocated by Doctors John Hunter and Virginia Alun Jones, contains numerous foods which are not useful in achieving optimal health. Still, I mention the diet because of the whole foods which it excludes. Certain whole foods can, in some people, create serious health problems. Here are some of the conditions caused by food intolerance: irritable bowel syndrome, migraine headache, asthma, rhinitis, gluten sensitive enteropathy, eczema, urticaria, cow's milk sensitive enteropathy, Crohn's disease, some types of arthritis, and hyperactivity in children.[7]

Perhaps one of the most troublesome symptoms of a food sensitivity is drowsiness and extreme fatigue. There are many causes for those two problems. Many people experience fatigue after eating because they have consumed a high-fat meal. I discovered the work by Hunter and Jones, a full year after my "health crisis" in 1992. At that time, I still experienced occasional bouts of fatigue, especially after meals. As I examined the exclusion diet, I realized that there were only two foods on their "not allowed" list which were part of my diet at that time—nuts and potatoes. I ate nuts only occasionally when we traveled by car, but I ate potatoes often. I eliminated both of those foods and then added them back one at a time. It was obvious that both foods caused me to experience fatigue and exhaustion. Once I removed them from my diet, I no longer had any difficulty.

The foods which are "not allowed" on the Exclusion Diet are best considered by categories:[8]

Meat: preserved meats, bacon, sausages

Fish: smoked fish, shellfish

Vegetables: potatoes, onions, corn

Fruit: citrus fruits, such as oranges, grapefruit

Cereals: wheat, oats, barley, rye, corn

Cooking oils: corn oil, vegetable oil (olive, soy, sunflower, and safflower oil allowed)

Dairy Products: cow's milk, butter, most margarines, cow's milk yogurt and cheese, eggs (goat's milk products allowed)

Beverages: coffee and tea, soft drinks, orange juice, grapefruit juice, alcohol, tap water

Miscellaneous: chocolate, yeast, preservatives, nuts

Dr. William G. Crook's Diet to Relieve Candida

The late Roger Williams, Ph.D., University of Texas, developed the concept of biochemical individuality. After we learn which foods are the most powerful, we need to listen to our bodies and learn to make decisions about the foods, whole foods concentrates, and supplements we consume. Those of us who have experienced candida with its wide range of symptoms know that each individual must learn what his or her body needs. Dr. William G. Crook has rescued many with his dietary suggestions for those suffering from candida. Although his international best seller, *The Yeast Connection,* provides essential information, his more recent work, *The Yeast Connection Cookbook,* offers much better advice to those interested in building better health through nutrition. He discusses the nutritional value of many foods and addresses the problem of contaminants and additives in our foods supply. He understands completely which foods aggravate candida-related complexes.

Dr. Crook suggests that those suffering from candida-related illnesses begin with a trial diet. His experience has been that people who are suffering from candida-related illnesses are bothered by other sensitivities as well. The trial diet includes those foods which are most easily tolerated by people who suffer from food allergies and candida-related diseases:[9]

Vegetables: all except corn and peas

Legumes: none

Meats: all except bacon, sausage, hot dogs, or luncheon meats

Special crackers and bread: any which contain no wheat, rye, or corn

Beverages: filtered or distilled water

Miscellaneous: fresh shelled, unprocessed nuts, seeds and oils—no peanuts or pistachios

The diet excludes:[10]

All dairy products

Eggs and egg-containing products

Wheat or rye—or any foods containing them

Corn—or any foods containing it

Fruits—and any food containing fruit

Sugar—and any food containing sugar

Chocolate and colas

Yeast and any food containing yeast

Coffee and alcohol

Soy, peanuts, beans, and other legumes

Coloring and other additives

Fermented foods—miso, tamari, tempeh

All of these dietary regimes have been used success-fully to treat people with specific diseases. They are worth noting, not because any one person has everything figured out, but because each success contributes to our under-standing. We need to bow our knees and seek His guid-ance in this and all other issues of life.

Most of the foods which I consider the "power foods" are foods which appear on all of the lists of "foods to eat" which we have just outlined. Phase One "power foods" are those foods recommended by all of the physicians we have just discussed as part of their cure and treatment for spe-cific disorders. Phase Two "power foods" include vital, life-giving foods which we should add one by one as our bod-ies are able to tolerate them. Phase Three—whole foods which may cause problems are nutritious foods which are not tolerated by a great many people. These foods can be useful, but they are not essential for optimal health. We should avoid them if we have any illness or disease—and remember, obesity is a disease. These foods are not the ones we should include while our bodies are in a weakened state. Some people will need to avoid one or more of these foods forever in order to maintain optimal health. We need to understand our "biochemical individuality" and praise God for the foods which heal and sustain us. These simple categories help us remember the research concern-ing food in a way which best answers the question, "What should I eat?" Phase One power foods are foods which enable us to make a giant leap forward as we seek optimal health. These foods are the ones which are best able to prevent and cure degenerative disease.

Phase One Power Foods—the Essentials

Green Leafy Vegetables: Greens have a high content of chlorophyll, carotenoids, calcium, iron, magnesium, manganese, potassium, vitamin A, and vitamin C. They provide a rich source of omega-3 fatty acids. We can drink our greens by juicing them with a masticating juicer which breaks up the cells and fibers of the food and gives us optimal nutritional value. Or, we can eat a number of greens cooked. For simple preparation we can use stainless steel, waterless cookware, or a steamer. Many greens are most delightful served raw in salads. However we serve them, greens are an important source of omega-3 fatty acids. Many people following whole foods regimes do not get a sufficient amount of this nutrient.

Salad Greens: Belgian endive, butterhead, chicory, crisphead, escarole and endive, loose-leaf lettuce, mache, parsley, romaine, sorrel, spinach, swiss chard, and watercress.

Cooked Greens: beet greens, collards, dandelion greens, kale, mustard, and turnip greens.

Cruciferous Vegetables: These are powerful in preventing and curing heart disease and cancer. We should consume a minimum of three one-cup servings each day. For optimal health, we can easily consume much more. Vegetables in this group are broccoli, kohlrabi, cauliflower, kale, turnip, radishes, rutabaga, cabbage, watercress, brussels sprouts, mustard greens, and horseradish.

Other Phase One Vegetables: asparagus, green beans, beets, carrots, celery, chard, okra, and yams.

Fruits: avocado. In spite of the high fat content of this food, it is excellent in building health. Avocados are very good for hypoglycemics because they stabilize blood sugar levels. This fruit has more potassium than bananas. The oil contains vitamins A, D, E, and fourteen minerals.

No fruits other than the avocado are appropriate for Phase One. Fruits quickly convert to simple sugars in the

body and often promote yeast infections. They are de-
stabilizing for hypoglycemics and diabetics. As we grow
stronger, fruits are added one at a time in Phase Two.
Again, we are individuals biochemically. We will know how
well we tolerate fruit by the way we feel. Headaches, fatigue, or shakiness indicate that we are not tolerating fruit
well at all. I suggest that no one begin eating fruits as long
as they are obese. When we are obese, our bodies are
weakened and stressed. Vegetables, vegetable juices, and
water can be used to cleanse our bodies. When we "crave"
fruit, it is because we are craving the fruit sugar. If we eat
grain and extra virgin olive oil, that craving will cease. The
lack of fruit in Phase One is often an important factor in
weight loss because many people who are overweight are
also hypoglycemic. Fruits are among those "healthy" foods
that actually contribute to obesity. The avocado, on the
other hand, is a "high-fat" food that helps us lose weight.

Grain: Amaranth, buckwheat, and quinoa are usually
tolerated by those who are allergic to various cereal grains.
Dr. Crook recommends that patients buy them in small
quantities until they determine whether or not they can
tolerate them. Although I enjoy all grains, the grain which
I believe is the supreme "power food" is spelt. I can truly
say that when I began eating spelt instead of brown rice,
I grew stronger and more energetic. Having eaten brown
rice for a number of years, perhaps my body needed relief
from the monotony. Those who are sensitive to cereal
grains can tolerate spelt better than any other grain. In
comparison to wheat, spelt has more crude fiber and is
higher in protein. Spelt is cooked differently than rice,
amaranth, quinoa, and buckwheat. Simply put the spelt in
a pot and cover it with water, one inch above the grain. Let
the spelt soak in the water overnight. Then bring the spelt
to a boil; after it reaches a boil, turn the pot on the lowest
setting and cook the spelt for one hour. The grain will be
soft and tender, but firm. The water never makes the spelt
mushy. The texture itself makes the grain ideal for hot or
cold salads.

One of the things I learned from the macrobiotic healing system is the value of intact grains. Not only are they essential for hypoglycemics and diabetics, they are essential for anyone who is in a weakened state. The intact grains (i.e., the whole grain before it is flaked or milled) promotes a steady blood sugar level. This is essential for gaining strength and energy.

We can add the other grains and flour products from Phase Three when our bodies are well and strong. Freshly milled flour—consumed by people who are well and whose diet consists of intact grains, legumes, vegetables, and fruits (if desired)—is a useful and healthful product.

Essential Fats: As we discussed in Step Two, flaxseed oil is the richest source of omega-3 fatty acids. Those who do not consume a large amount of greens daily need to take a tablespoon of flaxseed oil every day. This is wisdom. As we mentioned earlier, many of the contemporary degenerative diseases are the result of essential fatty acid deficiencies.

Extra virgin olive oil is a powerful, life-giving food. Experts now believe that unrefined, extra virgin olive oil contributes significantly to longevity. Olive oil reduces the effects of aging by protecting the tissues and organs of our bodies, as well as protecting the brain. Not only does olive oil reduce gastric acidity, it protects us against ulcers and helps food pass through the intestines. Olive oil improves the level of High Density Lipoproteins (HDL), the good cholesterol, and reduces the build-up of Low-Density Lipoproteins (LDL), the bad cholesterol.

Phase One is a place for everyone to begin. It is also a place to go when our bodies are weak and overworked. These grains and vegetables and one fruit (avocado) provide a variety of tastes, textures, and colors. We can juice a great quantity of our vegetables or juice none of them. Those who are battling a disease do well to include juicing in their regime. Juices therapy saves lives. Books about juicing abound. The life of Dr. Norman Walker has been an inspiration to many. He had a serious illness in his fifties. He regained his health by drinking raw fruit and vegetable juices. His diet consisted of raw foods and he lived to be 119. Dr. Walker wrote his last book at the age of 115. The value of Dr. Walker's regime ought to be carefully considered as we listen to our own bodies.

Some people who begin Phase One will be able and anxious to consume all of the vegetables raw in order to rebuild and rejuvenate their bodies as quickly as possible. Others will not be able to tolerate such a regime; the cleansing action may be too harsh or their digestive systems may not be able to handle a large amount of raw food initially. Clinics in the United States and Mexico use raw vegetable juice therapy in curing diseases which are pronounced "incurable" by medical doctors in the United States and elsewhere. Asthma, arthritis, bone cancer, brain cancer, breast cancer, colon cancer, diabetes, emphysema, liver cancer, lung cancer, lupus, lymphoma, and multiple sclerosis are only a few of the long list of diseases which have been and are being cured by raw juice therapy. Often, as we will discuss later, raw juices are used in conjunction with other nutritional therapies.

My own diet consists almost entirely of Phase One foods. The Phase Two foods which I eat regularly are a variety of legumes, onions, and garlic. I also eat wedges of apple from time to time. Although fruits offer nutritional advantages, I do well only with apples occasionally. I eat intact grains almost exclusively. For a treat, I make a delicious flatbread from freshly milled spelt flour, water, sea salt, and grated carrots. I use no leavening and no other ingredients; even people who are accustomed to eating processed, devitalized foods find this flatbread delightful. My morning and afternoon meals are usually raw, unless the weather is quite cold; then I consume some cooked vegetables both in the afternoon and early evening. I use sea salt to season my food—with no ill effects. By the grace and mercy of God, I no longer experience hypoglycemic episodes. I am strong, well, and at my ideal weight. I am thankful for the delicious array of foods He has provided.

As I will mention later in this chapter, I rely on whole foods concentrates as my "juice therapy." As I will explain, these foods have changed our lives.

My husband, Gary, has a very different regime. He drinks raw, organic carrot juice for breakfast and before his evening meal. He eats a raw fruit lunch (apples and bananas usually) and enjoys a large green salad with grains in the mid-afternoon. In the evening, he eats both raw and cooked vegetables. With that meal, he enjoys pasta or bread made from freshly milled flour. Gary has always been strong and fit. He is able to benefit from a variety of foods in Phase One, Phase Two, and Phase Three. Absolutely nothing—Phase One, Phase Two, Phase Three, or Phase "Junk"—bothers him. We all know these people; they are biochemical "mysteries." Initially, they may not be sensitive to the limitations of others. I encourage people all the time who have spouses who cannot understand their physical weaknesses in regard to food. My advice is this: attend to gaining strength as God gives you wisdom and discipline. Only by faith are we able to see the power of God about to be perfected in our weaknesses. It is only by the Spirit of God that any of us have ears to hear the Word of our Lord who says: "My grace is sufficient for you, for power is perfected in weakness" (2 Cor. 12:9). When we have physical limitations and find ways to overcome afflictions through His Word and wisdom, we become an encouragement to our families, friends and, acquaintances. When we rely on His support, we trust Him to move on the hearts of those around us. He is truly our "hiding place."

> Thou art my hiding place; Thou dost preserve me from trouble;
>
> Thou dost surround me with songs of deliverance.
>
> I will instruct you and teach you in the way which you should go;
>
> I will counsel you with my eye upon you.
>
> Do not be as a horse or as the mule which have no understanding.

Whose trappings include bit and bridle to hold
them in check,

Otherwise they will not come near to you.

Many are the sorrows of the wicked;

But he who trusts in the Lord, lovingkindness shall
surround him.

Be glad in the Lord, and rejoice you righteous ones,

And shout for joy all you who are upright in heart.
(Ps. 32:7–11)

Phase Two Power Foods

Phase Two power foods should be added one at a time
and consumed as we are able to tolerate them.

Legumes: These are important foods for reasons we
have discussed in Step Two. Many people who suffer with
candida-related illnesses cannot tolerate them until their
bodies are stronger. Begin slowly and rotate the types of
beans which you consume.

Vegetables: garlic, onions, peas, beans, and seeds.

Garlic is a wonder food and should be eaten as soon
as we are able to tolerate it. Some people will have no
difficulty with garlic even as they begin Phase One; this is
most fortunate, because garlic heals and revitalizes our
bodies. Garlic often stops symptoms in patients with candida-related complex. However, those who have food sensitivities often suffer allergic reactions when they eat garlic.
If we cannot tolerate certain foods, we need to go back to
Phase One until we gain strength; then try again.

Garlic has been proven effective in treating a wide
range of diseases. Those who suffer from pulmonary disorders actually find healing from asthma, bronchitis, and
pneumonia. Garlic is so powerful an antimicrobial that it
has been effectively used to treat at least eight types of
antibiotic resistant bacteria.[11] Those with gastrointestinal
disorders such as colitis find total relief when they begin
using fresh garlic. Allergies, arthritis, arteriosclerosis, can-

cer, diabetes, and hypoglycemia have all been treated effectively with garlic.

Onions are from the same family as garlic. Garlic and onions contain phytochemicals called allytic sulfides that research studies indicate may be useful in preventing stomach cancer. The phytochemicals issue a wake-up call to the enzymes inside the cells which have the ability to detoxify cancer-causing chemicals. They are also cleansers for our blood. As soon as we can tolerate them, we should eat them.

All vegetables except the nightshade family should be added in Phase Two. Peas and all freshly sprouted beans and seeds ought to be included at this time, as well as garlic and onions. Add them one at a time in order to understand which foods, if any, cause problems. Fatigue and sluggishness are subtle but significant indications that we can't tolerate a particular food. Other symptoms of food sensitivities are more severe. We will discuss the reasons why some people must avoid the nightshade vegetables later. These vegetables are among the most popular foods: tomatoes, potatoes, eggplant, and peppers (green, red, chili, paprika, cayenne). Tobacco is a member of this family.

Grains: Patients with celiac sprue (an intolerance to gluten) cannot tolerate the gluten present in wheat, oats, barley, rye, and triticale (a cross between wheat and rye). Symptoms of gluten intolerance range from bloating, gas, pain, and bouts of diarrhea to burning blisters, bumps, and lesions. People with candida-related complex usually cannot tolerate wheat and corn. Therefore, all grains except wheat, rye, oats, barley, triticale, and corn ought to be included.

Grains to include one at a time are brown rice, kamut, millet, sorghum. (Phase One already includes amaranth, quinoa, and spelt.) Those who have no concern about sensitivities to the glutenous grains and corn may wish to add them at this time.

People who have been diagnosed as wheat sensitive often find that when they cook the wheat berries or consume freshly milled wheat flour, they have no problems. I have personally talked to numbers of parents whose children fall into this category. Certainly, people should try the whole food product before concluding that they are sensitive to a specific grain; the processing, instead of the specific food, may be the problem.

Freshly milled grain flours: It is best to eat the intact grain first. If the grain is tolerated when it is consumed "intact," then it is wise to mill that particular grain. Sometimes we get weak eating too much flour, and we need to return to the intact grain.

Fruits: Those who are able to tolerate fruits or fruits in moderation should add all of the fruits except citrus. (Also omit tomatoes which are part of the nightshade family.)

Fermented foods: Miso and tempeh are fermented foods made from soy or grains. They are excellent sources of B12. As soon as these products can be tolerated they should be added to the diet. Tamari sauce is naturally fermented and preserved and should be used instead of commercial soy sauce.

Phase Three Whole Foods That Are Not Power Foods

Many of these foods contain important nutrients and make important contributions to the diets of many. But, some of the foods in this category are harmful to a great many people. None of the foods in this group are essential for optimal health, but they are included here because they are life-enhancing for many people.

Dehydrated foods: These foods provide convenience and nutrition in an acceptable form if the foods are dehydrated at home and do not contain harmful preservatives.

Nuts, seeds, and sweeteners: We need to spend our fat grams on the foods which are essential for optimal health. If we eat the essential fats, the healthy fats, we get thin; if we eat other fats and oils, we get fat. If we are at our ideal weight and if our cholesterol is 150 or below, there may be a place for a few freshly shelled raw nuts and seeds in our diets. We need first to get our fats from beans, grains, fruit, and vegetables. Extra virgin olive oil and flaxseed oil are the very best sources of fat.

For many people, life is unbearable without sweeteners. For those people, I hope that the sweeteners which I list in the whole foods pantry (Step Two) are satisfactory. Grain sweeteners, fruit juice concentrates, and even honey are acceptable for many people. They ought to be consumed in moderation.

Many people who are tired, obese, and plagued by headaches simply need to get off all sweeteners and fruit until they are totally well. I know diabetics and borderline diabetics who will not give up these foods. Although they feel badly after eating simple sugars, they are unable to stop. They continue to weaken their bodies and to risk serious illness. They are in bondage. All of us are weak in some area, but until we recognize our bondage and submit our will to Him, we cannot get free. And, getting free in Christ is more thrilling than any pleasure the enemy may be using to cause us temptation. Christ is greater than the tempter. If we ask Him for the grace to walk in wisdom, we will discover that our senses are truly renewed. Gradually, we will awaken to the taste, texture, and beauty of vegetables and grains. His provision is wonderful.

Our children often ask me, as they are eating muffins sweetened with fruit juice or a bowl of fruit, if I mind not eating those things.

My answer is this: I would like to eat fruits and naturally sweetened foods, and I remember the tastes of those foods very well; but I have developed new tastes. I am satisfied with the foods I eat, and I am unspeakably grateful to God that I am well. I think that the key to all of our limitations, whatever they may be, is this: the privilege of being alive is more important than anything.

Every person who is hypoglycemic, diabetic, and/or obese needs to live on the foods listed in Phase One and stay with those foods until they are well.

The nightshade family: Before I discuss the wonderful benefits we may receive from tomatoes, potatoes, peppers (green, red, chili, paprika, cayenne, hot, sweet), and eggplant, we need to examine the unpleasant effects these foods often have on our bodies. The nightshades are high in alkaloids. These chemical substances effect us physiologically. Although like proteins they have a high nitrogen content, they are unlike proteins in that they are not tissue builders. Rather they are stimulants, hallucinogens, medicines, and poisons. Well-known alkaloids are caffeine (in coffee), theobromine (in chocolate), as well as opium, heroin, morphine, strychnine, and quinine. These alkaloids are present in all parts of the nightshade foods. Peppers, tomatoes, and eggplants have only trace amounts. Potatoes contain the alkaloid solanine, which is most abundant under the skin. If potatoes are stored under light and heat, the solanine reaches toxic levels. Nightshades cause serious problems for many people because they cause the body to deposit calcium (bone matter) in inappropriate places. The alkaloids in potatoes and tomatoes pull calcium out of the blood and bones. When too much calcium is liberated, the excess is redeposited in soft tissues as spurs, stones, plaque, or other calcifications. This phenomenon is often the cause of many degenerative diseases; among them are hypertension, lupus erythmatosis, arthritis, arteriosclerosis, coronary disease, cerebral sclerosis, osteoporosis, chronic bronchitis, rheumatoid arthritis, and kidney stones. Some health practitioners advise their arthritic patients not to eat even traces of the nightshade foods—potato flour, paprika, cayenne, hot peppers—found in processed foods or condiments (e.g., Tabasco).[12]

> People who have followed these suggestions report good results, including remissions of arthritic pain, rheumatoid arthritis, osteoarthritis, bursitis, tennis elbow, gout, lower-back pain, headaches, high blood pressure and a host of related conditions.[13]

The effectiveness in curing arthritis by eliminating nightshades from the diet has been well documented. It is important that we recognize the problems associated with these foods as well as the benefits they have to offer. Before we move on to a discussion concerning the nutritional advantages offered by potatoes, tomatoes, eggplant, and peppers, we need to mention one more disadvantage regarding potatoes. They cause a rapid rise in insulin and blood sugar levels which presents a problem for diabetics and hypoglycemics. I noticed a wonderful improvement in my own stamina when I quit eating potatoes; the effect on the blood sugar may well be the reason. People who are overweight frequently have problems with diabetes or low blood sugar. I suggest that they eliminate the nightshades until they reach optimal weight. Many people find it quite disturbing to think of giving up potatoes. Dieters often eat a lot of potatoes, but this is not wise. A quick rise in insulin and blood sugar may be tolerable for those who are strong and well, but it is not good for those who are obese.

And, now the good points: eggplant has a reputation for enhancing immunity and preventing atherosclerosis. Potatoes are actually described by some nutritionists as a nearly perfect food. Potatoes contain high amounts of vitamins A, B, C, and are rich in vitamins and minerals. Potato skins have the greatest amount of nutrients, but if the skins are green they contain solanine. As we discussed earlier, solanine is a toxic chemical which potatoes produce when they are exposed to light. Scientists at Cornell University reported in 1994 that two of the estimated ten thousand phytochemicals which are present in tomatoes wipe out the formation of cancer-causing substances.[14] Tomatoes are high in lycopene which is another type of carotene. Scientists believe that is the explanation for studies which indicate that consuming tomatoes offers protection against cancer. Peppers are another nightshade offering important benefits. Hot chili peppers contain the phytochemical capsaicin which prevents lung and other cancers. Cayenne pepper is used for circulation and heart disorders. Externally, it is used in cream form to relieve arthritic pain.

Conclusion Regarding Power Foods

We each have a different biochemical makeup. The final responsibility is ours. We need to listen to our bodies and seek the wisdom of the Lord. By restricting our diets to Phase One power foods, we are not entering a state of deprivation, but, rather, we are giving our bodies the opportunity to benefit from the powerful foods which exist.

The Dehydrated Green Juice of Young Barley Leaves: God's Miracle Food

As I mentioned in Part One, I struggled for two years with pharyngeal spasms. During that time, I did everything I knew to do in terms of diet and discipline. I sought the Lord's help in learning to be quiet and to trust Him. I still seek His help in those areas and He continues to teach me. I know that in regard to the spasms, He mercifully provided a way of escape.

After having consumed nutritional supplements for twenty years and having used isolated nutrients for that long, I did not think of whole food concentrates as being "powerful." I considered megavitamins to be a short cut to healing and health, in combination with an excellent whole foods regimen. Then, early in July of 1994, I felt impressed to try the whole food concentrate that a friend recommended. She assured me that the maltodextrin in the product would not bother hypoglycemics or diabetics. But, I realized that I could only be certain of that after trying it. In the early printings of this manuscript, I mentioned that the maltodextrin had no adverse effect on my blood sugar level. Since that was the only barley product of its kind on the market at that time, I was more than willing to consume this green food in spite of the fact that it contained maltodextrin. Then, after two weeks, I realized that I had not had a pharyngeal spasm since I began taking the green juice concentrate. In August, I increased my dosage to one tablespoon, three times a day. Within weeks I no longer needed to eat breakfast immediately upon arising. After I awoke, I drank the green powder mixed in water, and I did not care to eat my first meal until mid-morning or noon. I experienced a better-than-caffeine lift and no side effects. For the first time in over twenty years, I was able to fast! My husband had no interest in the product until he saw the changes in my life. Then, he began taking one tablespoon, three times a day. Now we both realize that in green barley juice we have one of the most important single sources of essential nutrients available anywhere.

Yoshihide Hagiwara, M.D., often described as one of the most knowledgeable and honored pharmacologists in Japan, discovered the life-enhancing benefits of green barley grass and produced the world's first green juice product. Learning how to capture the nutrients in a usable product required extensive research. His spray-drying process has been patented in Japan, the United States and many other countries.

When this book first went to press, there were no other products which I considered comparable to those manufactured using Dr. Hagiwara's patented process. At this writing, however, I must advise readers of changes in the green foods market and make my recommendations based on those changes. When I discovered that I could buy certified organically grown green barley juice manufactured by a process that requires no binders, fillers, sweeteners or additives of any kind, I wanted that quality product for myself, for my family and friends, and for those who have read my recommendations and sought my advice. I first learned about this new green barley extract in 1996 while I was a guest on a network radio show; during the commercial break, I heard an advertisement about certified organically grown green barley juice, processed "on site" using vacuum dehydration. I discovered that unlike the green juice which I used and recommended, the product manufactured by GKC International contains 100% green barley leaf extract. Their dehydration process does not require the use of maltodextrin and their product contains no binders, no fillers, no sweeteners and no additives of any kind. The green barley extract used by GKC International is processed at 88 degrees Fahrenheit to lock in nutritional potency.

As a result of the advertisement that I heard, I began researching the changes in the green foods market and verifying the claims made by GKC International. Finally, we had a number of lengthy discussions on the telephone with the president and CEO of GKC International and later, during the summer of 1996, my husband, Gary, and I met with him to discuss formulating our own products. That summer Gary developed a business plan for the company which has become Green Pastures. The company was funded in August 1996 by a man and wife who became our friends through the book, *Health Begins In Him*, and through the seminar, Health Begins In Him (which they sponsored in their city). Gary operates Green Pastures and serves as president and CEO. Our mission is simply to provide whole foods, whole food concentrates and nutraceuticals which are of superior quality. We offer documentation verifying that our products are certified organic. We fully disclose each ingredient, and the percentage of each ingredient, on our labels.

We have walked on a few of the several thousand acres in southern Utah on which our certified organic green barley and other cereal grasses are grown. We have enjoyed fellowship with the man who grows the crops and processes the cereal grasses which we use in our products. The green barley grass and alfalfa grass contained in our unique formulations are certified organically grown at an elevation of over 5,000 feet, in the mineral rich soil of an ancient volcanic bed. Green Pastures has spent thousands of dollars on laboratory tests which compare our products with the market leaders. We publish the results of tests conducted by well-known and highly respected independent laboratories in order to substantiate our claims. Consumers have responded to our message concerning organic farming methods: if the nutrients are not in the soil, they will not be in the plants—and plants are our most important source of vital nutrients!

Barley Harvest, Carrots Plus, and Garden Wonder

Three products, each bottle containing 75 one tea-spoon servings, provide vitamins, minerals and amino acids which we need in order to achieve or maintain optimal health. All of us would do well to eat platters of certified organic carrots, raw broccoli, cauliflower, parsley, kale, and cabbage (red, green and purple) each day or to drink the juice, freshly extracted from them, each morning and night. The truth is that most people across America do not have access to a wide variety of organic vegetables; and many of those who do have access to organic food, find that extracting fresh vegetable juice each day, from one or many vegetables, demands too much of their time, money and energy. Juices from the organic cereal grasses—green barley leaves, green alfalfa leaves and oat grass leaves—are certainly not readily available in local markets. However, when these organically grown cereal grasses—as well as carrots, kale and cruciferous vegetables—are processed on site and dehydrated at 88 degrees Fahrenheit, as are ours, consumers receive all the live enzymes and micronutrients which are available in the freshly picked raw food.

Barley Harvest is 99.6% dehydrated green juice from certified organic young barley plants and contains .4% stevia, an herb which helps stabilize blood sugar levels and enhances the flavor of the green barley. Carrying agents such as maltodextrin are neither required nor used in the vacuum dehydration process which is used to produce our whole food concentrates.

Barley Harvest is highly effective in preventing, treating, and curing degenerative disease. It provides the essential balance of minerals which is the key to maintaining optimal health. Potassium in the living cells is the source of life activity. The standard American diet does not allow potassium and other minerals to remain in favorable balance. Barley Harvest gives us potassium, magnesium, calcium, iron, and phosphorus in perfect balance. As we have discussed, most diets contain an excess of phosphorus. (Phases One and Two "power foods" prevent that excess in phosphorus.) Some of the most nutritious foods are lacking in the important trace minerals manganese and zinc, both of which are present in significant amounts in Barley Harvest. The five essential nutrients—minerals, vitamins, enzymes, chlorophyll, and protein—are abundantly available in Barley Harvest. Barley Harvest contains whole complex vitamins in an active (natural), bioavailable form. For example, the nutrients in a crushed, raw vegetable are reduced by as much as half within a period of five minutes; as much as 70 percent of the nutrients are lost from the crushed, raw vegetable within twenty minutes. Vitamins are the essential nutrients which enable enzymes to function. This whole food concentrate offers us the most powerful supply of vitamins and minerals available anywhere.

Barley Harvest contains large amounts of both essential amino acids (valine, leucine, isoleucine, phenylalanine, threonine, and methionine) and the essential fatty acids—linoleic acid and linolenic acid—which are not synthesized in the human body. As we discussed in Step Two, many medical researchers and scientists agree that the rapid increase in degenerative diseases is in a great measure caused by a lack of the omega-3 fatty acids. Barley Harvest is a lifeline for those who eat devitalized food; it is a rejuvenator for those of us who enjoy a whole foods dietary regime.

The chlorophyll in green barley leaves enables our bodies to produce healthy hemoglobin. It is an anti-inflammatory and a germicide. By applying Barley Harvest topically we can heal severe skin inflammation and injury. It also works just as effectively—sufferers say "miraculously"—on peptic ulcers and gastritis. The deodorizing properties of chlorophyll are widely understood; now we have both a convenient and totally reliable source.

Finally, Barley Harvest offers us a convenient, ready supply of live enzymes. These enzymes are the regulators of the body. All of the chemical changes in our cells are made possible by enzyme activity. Since the natural enzymes are not destroyed in the vacuum dehydration process, we are able to benefit from the more than twenty enzymes found in green barley extract. When we fail to consume sufficient enzymes, our bodies become weak and the decomposition of fats fails to occur properly. As the fats build up, we gain excess weight. Obesity is a disease and a signal that our enzyme activity is insufficient. Raw foods and certified organic whole food concentrates restore enzyme activity.

Carrots Plus contains 60% certified organic vacuum dehydrated carrots and 39.6% premium deoiled soybean lecithin (characterized by its high phospholipid concentration). The body can absorb only 1% of the beta carotene in raw carrots. Cooking breaks down the fibrous walls of the carrot, increasing the absorption to 19%. However, our bodies can absorb virtually 100% of the beta carotene in vacuum dehydrated carrots. Most important, the vacuum dehydration process removes moisture in a fraction of the time that dehydration requires.

Carrots Plus is high in beta carotene, vitamin B complex, and vitamins C, D, E and K. It is also high in minerals: calcium, copper, magnesium, manganese, phosphorus, potassium, and sulphur. Studies show that the beta carotene in whole foods and whole food concentrates is useful in the prevention of cancer, heart attacks, strokes and cardiovascular disease. Foods rich in beta carotene are an essential part of a balanced diet. The great plus in Carrots Plus is the deoiled lecithin. Soy lecithin is high in choline and inositol. Studies indicate that lecithin is useful in helping the brain to function optimally, emulsifying fat and lowering cholesterol.

Garden Wonder is 60% dehydrated juice from certified organic cabbage (red, purple, green), kale, broccoli, parsley and cauliflower; it contains 30% dehydrated juice from certified organic alfalfa grass, 9.6% dehydrated juice from certified organic oat grass and .4% stevia. This cruciferous blend is high in cancer antidotes such as indoles, glucosinolates, and dithiolthiones. The chlorophyll, carotenoids, calcium and high mineral content of dark green vegetables heal the body and strengthen the immune system. Alfalfa contains biotin, folic acid, pantothenic acid, pyridoxine and vitamins A, B, C, D, E, K and U. It is an important source of calcium, phosphorous, magnesium, iron, selenium and zinc. Concentrated alfalfa is an excellent source of B12 and of silicon (a mineral which research indicates is important for the development of good teeth, hair and nails). This blend of cruciferous and dark green leafy vegetables, alfalfa, and oat grass makes Garden Wonder one of the most nutritionally dense whole food concentrates available.

Oral Hygiene: Preventing Gum Disease, Loss of Teeth, and Halitosis

The way that we eat is the most important single factor in preventing gum disease and loss of teeth. This chapter and Step Two offer the information which is essential in achieving optimal health. Healthy teeth and gums begin with a healthy body.

We know that we need to brush and floss our teeth after every meal or snack. But, many of our dentists have not recommended the most effective products for oral hygiene. It is now widely recognized that those mouth rinses which contain alcohol are a hazard to our health. There is a risk of oral cancer with prolonged use. The alcohol also softens the bonding agents. Toothpastes which are recommended by and distributed free of charge as samples are often lacking in the ingredients which are now recognized as most effective in soft tissue management.

Stabilized Chlorine Dioxide

This ingredient has been used to purify water by eliminating microorganisms for over fifty years. The EPA has tested this ingredient and recommends it over chlorine for use in water purification. Stabilized chlorine dioxide never breaks down into chlorine, but, rather, when it is activated, it initiates an oxidation reaction, producing a solution which is noncarcinogenic. Chlorine, on the other hand, as it reacts in water, releases trihalomethanes, which are known carcinogenic substances. Oxygene is a pure pharmaceutical grade product. Lockheed and McDonnell Douglas specify this particular form of stabilized chlorine dioxide for use in the purification of the drinking water on their commercial flights.

Twenty to Ninety Million People Suffer from Chronic Halitosis

According to a study published in the September 1994 issue of *Reader's Digest,* most people with bad breath do not suffer from gum disease as dentists have assumed. The *Reader's Digest* article describes in great detail the horror of chronic halitosis. Prior to reading the article, I would have suggested that any sufferer 1) change to the kind of dietary regime recommended here, 2) take fiber supplements to cleanse the colon, 3) drink products containing chlorophyll, 4) consume Barley Harvest and other whole food concentrates, and 5) take nutritional supplements such as natural vitamin C, natural vitamin E, chelated selenium, and coenzyme Q10 (extracted from plant sources, all natural and free from any additives or other ingredients). I would have been certain of that good advice. But, these sufferers can actually get immediate relief. And, although I would counsel them to take each of the five steps listed above, I would first tell them how to resolve the symptoms (halitosis) of the real problem (a state of degeneration within their bodies). People with chronic halitosis are handicapped because they cannot go about the business of their lives. The odor is so great that people cannot be near them without backing away or turning their heads and holding their noses.

As the *Reader's Digest* article points out, the mouth area is the source of 80 to 90 percent of bad breath. An enlightened group of dentists around the country understand what simple procedures and state-of-the-art dental care products are needed to prevent halitosis and gum disease. Volatile sulphur compounds (VSCs) grow on the back of the tongue like a thick carpet. All of us need to brush the backs of our tongues with toothpaste containing stabilized chlorine dioxide, the ingredient which oxidizes the VSCs. Every tongue should be a rosy pink color. Cleaning up our insides will take longer, but life must go on. These products also eliminate the odor of fresh garlic, onion—anything. The toothpaste and mouthrinse I recommend are manufactured by Oxyfresh of Spokane and contain oxygene which I have already described.

Find a dentist who is teachable or who already knows about this company and their products. Although the great majority of chronic halitosis is caused by VSCs on the back of the tongue, there are two other major causes: 1) bacteria on the edge of the gums which leads to periodontal disease; and 2) medical problems in the sinuses and the tonsils which causes odor and requires treatment. Healthcare professionals now have an objective way to measure and diagnose the problem. The Halimeter measures volatile sulphur compounds, the byproducts of rotting bacteria and gum tissue. The machine draws out a sample breath with a vacuum pump; the readings assist the healthcare professional in diagnosing the cause of the patient's halitosis. There are live seminars as well as a dental satellite network available for men and women who are interested in preventative dentistry. We need to be certain that the toothpaste and mouthrinse we use are safe and effective. For more information, see the Resource Guide.

Cancer Patients Find an Oasis of Hope

Those of us who have seen our loved ones go through the deceit and madness of cancer treatment in the United States can rejoice in the knowledge that God has raised up servants to be His healing hands. Those who have just discovered that a friend, a loved one, or they themselves have cancer can take heart; God is giving us eyes to see the provision which He has made available. Those who never imagined a credible alternative can discover for themselves that our bodies can be healed of cancer. Christ has made a provision. I would like to introduce three very special medical doctors: Ernesto Contreras, Sr., M.D., Francisco Contreras, M.D., and Ernesto Contreras, Jr., M.D. These men know the Lord. They are helping patients receive their healing. We need to examine what these men do (results). We need to know who these men are (credentials). And, we need to know how they have achieved results (treatment).

Results:

Recently, I sat with my husband and children and watched a videotape featuring patients of Ernesto Contreras, Sr., M.D. The occasion documented in this video seems very like a family reunion, more especially, the reunion of a very warm and close-knit family. One could never imagine this setting at any hospital in the United States. Some of the patients have returned annually for decades, just to share the blessing with others who have survived cancer. Although they had once been considered "terminally ill" in the United States, they have recovered completely and are cancer free. The video is a documentary of this reunion. Patients tell of their love and concern for the other patients and their esteem for the Drs. Contreras. After hearing over a dozen testimonies, my ten-year-old daughter said, "Mother, I thought most people die from cancer." I answered, "In this country, most of them do." Then my six-year-old said, "Why don't they go to that place," she pointed to the television, "they're not dead!" Gary and I had tears in our eyes. We thought of various family members who have died from cancer—cousins who died when they were young, middle-aged aunts, my father. Nearly every family has a list. As we continued to watch the video, we listened to those who had come to have treatments; others had come for an annual checkup. All had come to celebrate life—as survivors. They had no tomorrows according to medical doctors in the United States. Most had gone to the Hospital Ernesto Contreras after they had tried everything else. The people we watched are among the more than fifty thousand patients who have been treated at the Contreras Oasis of Hope. Most were referred to the hospital by a survivor.

As I watched the video, I thought of my father's surgery and cancer treatment. I recalled the days with him and with my family at one of the most famous hospitals in America. I thought of the many conversations with the surgeons and the oncologists. I thought of the blindness, the foolishness, and the pride that characterizes much of the medical establishment in America. Then, I thought of the many physicians who are changing, who want to lead people to optimal health, who don't want to walk in darkness as doctors of death. All of us who have experienced God's healing hand must share the light that He has given. It may be the very spark which lights the way for someone lost in the darkness of disease. I believe my father would want me to shout from the housetops that a place like the Contreras Hospital, Oasis of Hope, exists.

The Contreras Oasis of Hope publishes a list of patients from the United States who are willing to share their testimonies. The list states where the cancer began in each patient and gives a name, address, and telephone number. How very kind and generous of these people to open their lives to strangers as an encouragement. They are giving back what was given to them—life.

Credentials:

Ernesto Contreras, Sr., M.D. founded the Oasis of Hope. His practice began with a private office and grew steadily to become the Good Samaritan Hospital in 1963. The hospital is now a fifty-thousand-square-foot facility which overlooks the Pacific Ocean in Playas, Mexico, located twenty-five miles south of San Diego, California. Dr. Contreras, Sr., and his two sons are M.D.'s and have specialized in oncology. They are dedicated to the use of nontoxic treatment. Dr. Francisco Contreras received a special recognition for developing the technique for the installation of the permanent onphalo-portal catheter.

Dr. Ernesto Contreras' philosophy is that the Contreras' contribution to the healing of the individual is only 30 percent of the process. All of their research and expertise with the most advanced and successful treatments available, he counts as less than half of the effort involved in the healing. He believes that the patient and the companion make up 70 percent of the process. The patient undergoes a dramatic change, a rebirth, a renewing of the spirit and a cleansing of the body. The companion is encouraged to nurture, support, and love the patient who is in great need.

The Contreras research team has tested more than seventy-five substances and selectively uses those that have been successful in their hospital or in treatment centers worldwide. But, the treatments work because they are dependent upon the Spirit of God. On the first page of the hospital manual, the role of the body, the mind, and the spirit are distinguished; faith, hope and love are acknowledged as essential for life.

These men are servants of God. The Contreras Chapel has grown to become a one thousand-member church. Dr. Contreras, Sr., and his wife, Rita, lead a weekly devotional for their employees. They state on their hospital brochure that the Contreras and their patients and companions stand together in promoting a spiritual, Christ-centered environment. What an incredible, refreshing difference in medical care. They do not see patients as "victims" or "customers," but rather as partners in God's plan.

Treatment:

Every patient receives customized treatment which meets his or her specific needs. After thirty years experience, they conduct themselves as a research team, alert to the special needs of each individual. Most programs include some of the following treatments:

Laetrile; Enzymes; Megavitamin Therapy

Hydrazine Sulfate

Clordranate

Liver Regenerating Agents

Neurological Regenerating Agents

Immune Modulating Agents

Organic Foods

Shark Cartilage (100 percent pure)

Antioxidants

Ozone Therapy

Warburg Therapy

Hormone Therapy

Multidisciplinary Management by specialists in cases where intensive care is needed

Nontoxic treatment and a good diet rebuild the body's immune system. But, the Contreras team considers the patient's spiritual growth as the most significant factor in recovery. They say this of the treatment:

> The success of the Contreras therapies are due to a combined attack to the cancer cells with external and internal weapons. The external ones are a mixture of natural cytotoxic substances which are very effective and specific against cancer cells given orally and intravenously and through a catheter directly to the liver in cases of liver metastasis. The internal weapons use the immune system which is boostered by a special program of immune therapy.[15]

The Oasis of Hope will provide further information regarding every aspect of treatment. Each of the therapies warrants a full discussion. Their toll-free telephone number is 1-800-700-1850.

In Closing:

For some people the information in this chapter may be something of a review; for others, Steps One through Four are filled with new information—too much new information. For the latter group, I offer this suggestion. Review the material bit by bit. I have spent years walking this out; readers will also need to learn by doing. For the most part, I have provided vital information. If we prepare ourselves for each of the last four action steps, we will be able to take those steps. We will experience strength and vitality we have never known. Step Five is a prayer and a benediction.

Present Your Bodies a Living and Holy Sacrifice: a Prayer and a Benediction

Preparation:

Ask the Lord for a broken spirit and a contrite heart.

Cultivate faith.

In his book, *None of These Diseases*, S. I. McMillen, M.D., teaches that poor mental and physical health are the result of our carnal nature. At the conclusion of this Christian classic, he describes the struggle we face.

> It will give us pain to bid a final farewell to the carnal part of our natures which has given us a large share of life's so-called pleasures. It will mean giving up some of our habits, our friends, our practices and our ways of thinking. Let us face it squarely—it is a sorrowful experience to bid adieu to every worldly pleasure, friend and habit that God marks for dismissal. Yet it is not a dismissal of worthwhile joys and friends but of those born, like Ishmael outside of God's will for our lives.

> Jesus recognizes that we will feel some pain in giving up that which is carnal, but He promises that we will receive here and now one hundred times as much of the worthwhile. . . . We may shed some tears in saying farewell to the old life and its lure, but our grief will seem inconsequential moments later when we experience the exhilaration of His resurrection, life and power within us.[1]

As Christians, we can only walk in optimal health when we travel the subdued, contented journey of Romans, chapter twelve. Truly this is the answer to our prayer: "Thy Kingdom come, Thy will be done, on earth as it is in heaven" (Matt. 6:10).

The lives of other saints offer us examples of every possible physical circumstance. First, there are those who serve Him in spite of physical weaknesses and handicaps. By His grace, those limitations do not hinder His work in their lives or rob them of joy. Second, there are those who have learned by His grace to care nothing about their physical well-being, in so far as they might be tempted to seek a life which assured them any measure of comfort; they live only in the hope of His Kingdom. This second group is recorded in Hebrews 11:35–38:

> And others were tortured, not accepting their release, in order that they might obtain a better resurrection; and others experienced mockings and scourgings, yes, also chains and imprisonment.

> They were stoned, they were sawn in two, they were tempted, they were put to death with the sword; they went about in sheepskins, being destitute, afflicted, ill-treated (men of whom the world was not worthy), wandering in deserts and mountains and caves and holes in the ground.

These men and women walked in the power of the Resurrection which transcended their physical circumstances. They lived with all of their being—mental, physical, and spiritual—in the abundant life which His Word promises we may obtain.

A third group of saints walk in a spirit of contentment and experience physical stamina which are not of this world. They receive blessings provided by God which further His Kingdom. One such saint, the record of whose life continues to bless me almost daily, is John Wesley. I find excerpts from his journals and biographical accounts of his life to be a source of constant encouragement. He lead an active life into his eighties, constantly riding on horseback and preaching as vigorously as ever at that time. He exercised extreme discipline and moderation in his daily diet, but his diet cannot possibly account for his exhilaration and stamina. His journals also record what we would call "a miraculous healing."

> 1746. Monday, March 17.—I took my leave of Newcastle and set out with Mr. Downes and Mr. Shepherd. But when we came to Smelton, Mr. Downes was so ill that he could go no further. When Mr. Shepherd and I left Smelton, my horse was so exceedingly lame that I was afraid I must have lain by too. We could not discern what it was that was amiss; and yet he would scarcely set his foot to the ground. By riding thus seven miles, I was thoroughly tired, and my head ached more than it had done for some months. (What I here aver is the naked fact: let every man account for it as he sees good.) I then thought, "Cannot God heal either man or beast, by any means, or without any?" Immediately my weariness and headache ceased, and my horse's lameness in the same instant. Nor did he halt any more either that day or the next. A very odd accident this also.[2]

Wesley had many accidents on horses and in stage coaches which resulted in no harm to him whatsoever. As we read Wesley's record of his daily life, we realize that this man of remarkable eloquence and genius could have achieved fame in literature or government. He chose to be a man of action in order that souls might receive the salvation of God. Biographers offer the testimonies of his contemporaries who witnessed the character of a man who walked in the faith and victory described and experienced by the Apostle Paul. In Wesley, we find a man who was not captured by circumstances—however hard or extraordinary. The pain of life never wounded his heart; his heart belonged to God. Aspects of his personality may seem to many of us to be odd, and his behavior often intransigent. Some of his responses and disciplines may appear harsh and insensitive. And yet, the words and work and way of his life are those of a man yielded to God, a man who lived the abundant life which the Apostle Paul lived, described, and exhorted us to live. Through the lives of men and women of God—whether they have been long deceased or are yet living—we are reminded that His peace overcomes the world. Like all saints who have known or who know victory in Christ, John Wesley measured all things according to their eternal worth. His simple rule of life conforms—as did the journey of his life—to Romans, chapter twelve.

John Wesley's Rule

Do all the good you can,
By all the means you can,
In all the ways you can,
In all the places you can,
At all the times you can,
To all the people you can,
As long as ever you can.

May this simple rule—and the Word of God on which it is based—encourage our hearts and enable us to "prove what the will of God is, that which is good and acceptable and perfect" (Rom. 12:2).

A Broken and Contrite Heart

Make me know Thy Ways, O Lord;
Teach me Thy paths.
Lead me in Thy truth and teach me,
For Thou art the God of my salvation;
For Thee I wait all the day.
Remember, O Lord, Thy compassion and Thy
    lovingkindnesses,
For they have been from of old.
Do not remember the sins of my youth or my
    transgressions;
According to Thy lovingkindness remember Thou
    me,
For Thy goodness' sake, O Lord. (Ps. 25:4-7)
The sacrifices of God are a broken spirit:
A broken and a contrite heart, O God, Thou wilt
    not despise. (Ps. 51:17)

The Author and Finisher of Our Faith

Now faith is the assurance of things hoped for, the
conviction of things not seen.
For by faith men of old gained approval.
By faith we understand that the worlds were prepared by the word of God, so that what is seen
was not made out of things which are visible.
(Heb. 11:1-3)

So That We May Not Grow Weary and Lose Heart

Let us also lay aside every encumbrance, and the
sin which so easily entangles us, and let us run with
endurance the race that is set before us, fixing our
eyes on Jesus, the author and the perfecter of faith,
who for the joy set before Him endured the cross,
despising the shame, and has sat down at the right
hand of the throne of God. For consider Him who
has endured such hostility by sinners against Himself, so that you may not grow weary and lose heart.
(Heb. 12:1-3)

The Abundant Life and How We May Achieve It

I urge you therefore, brethren by the mercies of
God, to present your bodies a holy and living sacrifice, acceptable to God, which is your spiritual
service of worship.

And do not be conformed to this world, but be
transformed by the renewing of your mind, that
you may prove what the will of God is, that which
is good and acceptable and perfect.

For through the grace given to me I say to every
man among you not to think more highly of himself
than he ought to think; but to think so as to have
sound judgment, as God has allotted to each a
measure of faith.

For just as we have many members in one body and
all the members do not have the same function, so
we who are many are one body in Christ, and indi-
vidually members one of another.

And since we have gifts that differ according to the grace given to us, let each exercise them accordingly: if prophecy, according to the measure of his faith; if service, in his serving; or he who teaches, in his teaching; or he who exhorts, in his exhortation; he who gives, with liberality; he who leads, with diligence; he who shows mercy, with cheerfulness.

Let love be without hypocrisy. Abhor what is evil; cling to what is good;

Be devoted to one another in brotherly love; give preference to one another in honor; not lagging behind in diligence, fervent in spirit serving the Lord; rejoicing in hope, persevering in tribulation, devoted to prayer, contributing to the needs of the saints, practicing hospitality.

Bless those who persecute you; bless and curse not. Rejoice with those who rejoice, and weep with those who weep.

Be of the same mind toward one another; do not be haughty in mind, but associate with the lowly. Do not be wise in your own estimation.

Never pay back evil for evil to anyone. Respect what is right in the sight of all men.

If possible, so far as it depends on you, be at peace with all men.

Never take your own revenge, beloved, but leave room for the wrath of God, for it is written, "Vengeance is Mine, I Will Repay," says the Lord.

But if your enemy is hungry, feed him, and if he is thirsty, give him a drink, for in so doing you will heap burning coals upon his head.

Do not be overcome by evil, but overcome evil with good. (Rom. 12:1–21)

Notes

Part One

1. *The Shorter Catechism* (Grand Rapids, MI: Reformed Baptist Church, 1991), 1.

2. Harvey and Marilyn Diamond, *Fit For Life* (New York: Warner Books, 1985), 16.

3. Ibid., 53.

4. *Childcraft, The How and Why Library*, vol. 10 (Chicago: Field Enterprises Educational Corporation, 1949), 90.

5. *Childcraft, The How and Why Library*, vol. 15 (Chicago: Field Enterprises Educational Corporation, 1949), 264.

6. John T. Fodor, et al., *Keeping Healthy*, 3d ed. (River Forest, Il.: Laidlaw Brothers, 1980), 118.

7. Wilfred E. Shute and Harold J. Taub, *Vitamin E for Ailing and Healthy Hearts* (New York: Pyramid House, 1969), 61–64.

8. Neal Barnard, M.D., *Food for Life, How the New Four Food Groups Can Save Your Life* (New York: Crown Trade Paperbacks, 1993), 128.

9. Michio Kushi, *The Book of Macrobiotics, The Universal Way of Health and Happiness* (Tokyo, Japan: Japan Publications, Inc., 1977), 164.

10. Dr. Mary Ruth Swope, *What To Eat and What Not To Eat*, Speaking at a conference held by Charles and Francis Hunter. Video tape, sixty minutes. Distributed by Swope Enterprises, Inc. Phoenix, Az.

11. Teresa Ann Dorian, Ph.D., *Eating Better Program Guide* (Salt Lake City: Nutriflex, 1993), 1–89.

12. Barnard, *Food For Life*, 127.

13. Ibid.

14. Yoshihide Hagiwara, M.D., *Green Barley Essence* (New Canaan, Ct.: Keats Publishing, Inc., 1985).

15. Dr. Mary Ruth Swope, speaking to the congregation at Faith Outreach Center, San Antonio, Tx., 21 August 1994. Audio tape, sixty minutes. Distributed by Faith Outreach Center, San Antonio, TX.

16. Barnard, *Food For Life*, 151.

17. Ibid., 158.

Step One

1. S. I. McMillen, M.D., *None of These Diseases* (New York: Fleming H. Revell, 1963), 82.

2. Dean Ornish, M.D., *Dr. Dean Ornish's Program for Reversing Heart Disease; The Only System Scientifically Proven to Reverse Heart Disease Without Drugs or Surgery* (New York: Random House, 1990).

3. Dr. Mary Ruth Swope, speaking to the congregation at Faith Outreach Center, San Antonio, Tx., 21 August 1994. Audio tape, sixty minutes. Distributed by Faith Outreach Center, San Antonio, TX.

4. Dr. Alfred B. Smith, *Faithlift* (Greenville, S.C.: Praise Resources, 1990), 6.

Step Two

1. Neal Barnard, M.D., *Food For Life, How The New Four Food Groups Can Save Your Life* (New York: Crown Trade Paperbacks, 1993), xiv.

2. *Childcraft, The How and Why Library*, vol. 15 (Chicago: Field Enterprises Educational Corporation, 1972), 264.

3. *World Book Encyclopedia*, vol. 10 (Chicago: Field Enterprises Educational Corporation, 1965), 466–470.

4. Ibid., 468.

5. John T. Fodor, et al., *Keeping Healthy*, 3d ed. (River Forest, Il.: Laidlaw Brothers, 1980), 114–117.

6. Julius B. Richmond, M.D., Elenore T. Pounds, M.A., Irma B. Fricke, R.N., M.S., *Health and Growth 2* (Glenview, Il.: Scott, Foresman and Company, 1971), 97–112.

7. Ibid.

8. Foder, *Keeping Healthy*, 114–117.

9. Neal Barnard, M.D., *Food for Life, How the New Four Food Groups Can Save Your Life* (New York: Crown Trade Paperbacks, 1993), 9.

10. Ibid., 10.

11. Dean Ornish, M.D., *Eat More, Weigh Less* (New York: Harper Collins Publishers, 1993), 34.

12. Pamela Weintraub, "The Healthiest Diet in the World," *McCalls* (December 1992): 44.

13. Dean Ornish, M.D., *Dr. Dean Ornish's Program for Reversing Heart Disease; The Only System Scientifically Proven to Reverse Heart Disease Without Drugs or Surgery* (New York: Random House, 1990), inside front book jacket cover.

14. Ibid.

15. Ornish, *Eat More, Weigh Less*, 31.

16. Barnard, *Food For Life*, 26.

17. Ibid., 27–28.

18. Ornish, *Eat More, Weigh Less*, 28.

19. Richard A. Knox, "Children's Fatty Diets Cause Early Health Risks," *Spartanburg Herald-Journal* (11 September 1993): A1, A4.

20. Ibid.

21. Ibid.

22. Barnard, *Food For Life*, 35.

23. Ornish, *Reversing Heart Disease*, 257.

24. Ibid., 261.

25. Annemarie Colbin, *Food and Healing* (New York: Random House, 1986), 167.

26. Barnard, *Food For Life*, 56.

27. Ibid., 56.

28. Ibid., 152.

29. Ibid., 153.

30. Ibid., 69.

31. Phyllis Herman, "Fats—Telling the Good from the Bad," *Health News and Review*, vol. 3, no. 4, (1993): 14.

32. Harvey and Marilyn Diamond, *Fit For Life* (New York: Warner Books, 1985), 74.

33. Ornish, *Reversing Heart Disease*, 260.

34. "Strict Diet May Affect Amino Acids," *Spartanburg Herald Journal* (24 January 1994): C2.

35. Barnard, *Food For Life*, 11.

36. Norma S. Upson, *The Bean Cookbook* (Seattle, Wa.: Search Press, 1982), 1.

37. Phyllis A. Balch, C.N.C. and James F. Balch, M.D., *Prescription for Cooking and Dietary Wellness* (Greenfield, In.: P.A.B. Publishing, Inc., 1992), 51.

38. Colbin, *Food and Healing*, 171.

39. Upson, *The Bean Cookbook*, 10.

40. Sharon Begley, "Beyond Vitamins," *Newsweek* (25 April 1994): 45–48.

41. Ibid., 48.

42. Ibid., 49.

43. Colbin, *Food and Healing*, 171.

44. Ingeborg M. Johnston, C.N. and James R. Johnston, Ph.D., *Flax-seed Oil and the Power of Omega-3* (New Canaan, Ct.: Keat Publishing, 1990), 29.

45. Ibid., 25.

46. Ibid., 8.

47. Ibid., 18.

48. Herman, "Fats—Telling the Good from the Bad," 14.

49. Barnard, *Food For Life*, 36.

50. Ibid., 37.

51. Herman, "Fats—Telling the Good from the Bad," 14.

52. Peter Yudkin, M.D., *Sweet and Dangerous* (New York: Bantam Paperback, 1972), 1–37.

53. E.M. Abrahamson, M.D. and A.W. Pezet, *Body, Mind, and Sugar* (New York: Avon Books, 1951), 1–12.

54. Dr. Mary Ruth Swope, speaking to the congregation at Faith Outreach Center, San Antonio, Tx., 21 August 1994. Audio tape, sixty minutes. Distributed by Faith Outreach Center, San Antonio, TX.

55. Balch, *Cooking and Dietary Wellness*, 175.

56. Dr. Mary Ruth Swope, *Some Gold Nuggets in Nutrition* (Phoenix, Az.: National Preventive Health Services, 1994), 22.

57. Sang Whand, "Reverse Aging Not Science Fiction But Science Fact," (unpublished article, Miami, Fl.: 1990).

58. Hans Diehl, M.D., Audio-taped Speech, Loma Linda, Ca.

59. Francisco Contreras, M.D., of the Contreras Cancer Clinic in Tiajuana, Mexico, in a speech delivered before an audience at the AIM International Convention in 1990, taken from an audio tape.

60. Yoshihide Hagiwara, M.D., *Green Barley Essence* (New Canaan, Ct.: Keats Publishing, 1985), 9–10.

61. Beatrice Hunter, *Consumer Beware* (New York: Simon & Schuster, 1971), 347.

62. Dr. Mary Ruth Swope, *Some Gold Nuggets in Nutrition* (Phoenix, Az.: National Preventive Health Services, 1994), 23–25.

63. *FDA Consumer* (October 1980), 7.

64. Yoshihide Hagiwara, M.D., *Green Barley Essence* (New Canaan, Ct.: Keats Publishing, 1985), 17.

65. *The Healthy Cell Concept* (Nampa, Id.: AIM International, 1993), 23.

66. Ibid.

67. Jean Carper, "Your Food Pharmacy: Try Stewing, Boiling and Poaching" *Spartanburg Herald Journal* (26 March 1992): C2.

Step Three

1. Neal Barnard, M.D., *Food for Life, How the New Four Food Groups Can Save Your Life* (New York: Crown Trade Paperbacks, 1993), 29.

2. Ibid., 130.

3. Thom Leonard, *The Bread Book, A Natural Whole-Grain Seed to Loaf Approach to Real Bread* (Brookline, Ma.: East West Health Books, 1990), 35.

4. Ibid., 38.

5. Ibid., 37.

6. Teresa Ann Dorian, Ph.D., *Eating Better Program Guide* (Salt Lake City: Nutriflex, 1993), 30.

Step Four

1. Paul Hoversten, "Congress May Ease Water Rules," *USA Today* (28 July 1994): 1A.

2. "Study Water Not Up to Standards" *The Orlando Sentinel* (15 March 1994): A-3.

3. Linda Kanamine, "Under-treated water flows to 50 million," *USA Today* (28 July 1994): 5A.

4. Dean Ornish, M.D., *Dr. Dean Ornishes Program for Reversing Heart Disease; The Only System Scientifically Proven to Reverse Heart Disease Without Drugs or Surgery* (New York: Random House, 1990), 253–302.

5. Ibid., 279.

6. Collin H. Dong, M.D. and Jane Banks, *The Arthritic's Cookbook* (New York: Thomas Y. Cowell, 1973), 28–29.

7. John Hunter, M.D., et al., *Food Intolerance, Are The Foods You Eat Making You Sick?* (Tucson, Az.: The Body Press, 1986), 10.

8. Ibid., 19.

9. William G. Crook, M.D., and Marjorie Hunt Jones, R.N., *The Yeast Connection Cookbook, A Guide to Good Nutrition and Better Health* (Jackson, Tn.: Professional Books, 1989), 97–98.

10. Ibid., 97.

11. Rob McCaleb, "Garlic-Infection Fighter," *Better Nutrition* (August 1993): 46.

12. Annemarie Colbin, *Food and Healing*, (New York: Random House, 1986), 176–179.

13. Ibid., 178.

14. Sharon Begley, "Beyond Vitamins," *Newsweek* (25 April 1994): 48.

15. "Contreras Care Oasis of Hope," hospital bulletin distributed by the Contreras Hospital.

Step Five

1. S.I. McMillen, M.D., *None of These Diseases* (Old Tappan, N.J.: Fleming H. Revel Company, 1963), 147.

2. *The Journal of John Wesley*, ed. Percy Livingstone Parker, (Chicago: Moody Press, 1951), 146.

If you would like to receive (1) a copy of Dr. Terry Dorian's newsletter, "Healthy Living"; (2) information about her workshops and seminars; or (3) a copy of her resource guide

Call Toll-Free
1-800-295-3477

We welcome any comments from our readers. Feel free to write to us at the following address:

Editorial Department
Huntington House Publishers
P.O. Box 53788
Lafayette, LA 70505

ORDER THESE HUNTINGTON HOUSE BOOKS !

- *ADD—*
  Theresa Lamson 11.99
- *Alzheimer's—*
  Teresa Strecker, Ph.D. 11.99
- *Anyone Can Homeschool—*
  Terry Dorian & Zan Peters Tyler 10.99
- *The Assault—*
  Dale A. Berryhill 10.99
- *Beyond Political Correctness—*
  David Thibodaux 10.99
- *Bible Promises—*
  edited by David England 9.99
- *The Big Book—*
  edited by David England 14.99
- *Circle of Death—*
  Richmond Odom 10.99
- *Children No More—*
  Brenda Scott 12.99
- *Combat Ready—*
  Lynn Stanley 10.99
- *The Cookbook: Health Begins In Him—*
  Terry Dorian and Rita M. Thomas 14.99
- *The Dark Side of Freemasonry—*
  Ed Decker 10.99
- *Deadly Deception—*
  Shaw \ McKenney 9.99
- *The Demonic Roots of Globalism—*
  Gary Kah 10.99
- *Dinosaurs and the Bible—*
  David Unfred 12.99
  with Teacher's Guide 13.99
- *Do Angels Really Exist?—*
  David O. Dykes 10.99
- *En Route to Global Occupation—*
  Gary Kah 10.99
- *First Lady—*
  Peter and Timothy Flaherty 11.99
- *Gender Agenda—*
  Dale O'Leary 11.99
- *Getting Out/Abused Women—*
  Kathy Cawthon 10.99

- *Global Bondage—*
  Cliff Kincaid 10.99
- *Global Taxes for World Government—*
  Cliff Kincaid 14.99
- *Health Begins in Him—*
  Terry Dorian 10.99
- *Hidden Dangers of the Rainbow—*
  Constance Cumbey 10.99
- *High on Adventure I, II, and III—*
  Stephen Arrington 9.99
- *The Hound of Heaven—*
  Gordon MacDonald 12.99
- *How to be a Great Husband—*
  Tobias Jungreis 11.99
- *How to Homeschool (Yes, You!)—*
  Julia Toto 3.99
- **Inside the New Age Nightmare—*
  Randall Baer 10.99/2.99
- *A Jewish Conservative Looks at Pagan America—*
  Don Feder .... 10.99/21.99 HB
- *Journey into Darkness—*
  Stephen Arrington 10.99
- *Legacy Builders—*
  Jim Burton 11.99
- *The Liberal Contradiction—*
  Dale A. Berryhill 10.99
- *The Media Hates Conservatives—*
  Dale A. Berryhill 10.99
- *Out of Control—*
  Brenda Scott 10.99
- *Outcome-Based Education—*
  Peg Luksik & Pamela Hoffecker 10.99
- *Please Tell Me—*
  Tom McKenney 10.99
- *Political Correctness—*
  David Thibodaux 10.99
- *Revival: Its Principles and Personalities—*
  Winkie Pratney 10.99
- *Sammy: Dallas Detective—*
  Robin Hardy 9.99
- *To Grow By Readers (20/Set)—*
  Janet Friend 49.95

*Available in Salt Series

Available at bookstores everywhere or order direct from:
Huntington House Publishers • P.O. Box 53788
Lafayette, LA 70505
Send check/money order. For faster service use VISA/
MASTERCARD.
Call toll-free 1-800-749-4009.
Add: Freight and handling, $3.50 for
the first book ordered, and
$.50 for each additional book up to 5 books.

Order These Huntington House Books !

- America Betrayed—Marlin Maddoux. 7.99
- The Assault—Dale A. Berryhill 9.99
- Beyond Political Correctness—David Thibodaux 9.99
- The Best of HUMAN EVENTS—Edited by James C. Roberts 34.95
- Can Families Survive in Pagan America?—Samuel Dresner 15.99/31.99
- Circle of Death—Richmond Odom 9.99
- Combat Ready—Lynn Stanley 9.99
- Conservative, American & Jewish—Jacob Neusner 9.99
- The Dark Side of Freemasonry—Ed Decker 9.99
- The Demonic Roots of Globalism—Gary Kah 9.99
- Don't Touch That Dial—Barbara Hattemer & Robert Showers 9.99/19.99
- En Route to Global Occupation—Gary Kah 9.99
- *Exposing the AIDS Scandal—Dr. Paul Cameron .7.99/2.99
- Freud's War with God—Jack Wright, Jr. 7.99
- Goddess Earth—Samantha Smith 9.99
- Gays & Guns—John Eidsmoe 7.99/14.99
- Health Begins in Him—Terry Dorian 9.99
- Heresy Hunters—Jim Spencer 8.99
- Hidden Dangers of the Rainbow—Constance Cumbey .9.99
- High-Voltage Christianity—Michael Brown 9.99
- Homeless in America—Jeremy Reynalds 9.99
- How to Homeschool (Yes, You!)—Julia Toto 4.99
- Hungry for God—Larry E. Myers 9.99
- I Shot an Elephant in My Pajamas—Morrie Ryskind w/ John Roberts 12.99
- *Inside the New Age Nightmare—Randall Baer 9.99/2.99
- A Jewish Conservative Looks at Pagan America—Don Feder 9.99/19.99
- Journey into Darkness—Stephen Arrington 9.99
- Kinsey, Sex and Fraud—Dr. Judith A. Reisman & Edward Eichel 11.99
- The Liberal Contradiction—Dale A. Berryhill 9.99
- Legalized Gambling—John Eidsmoe 7.99
- Loyal Opposition—John Eidsmoe 8.99
- The Media Hates Conservatives—Dale A. Berryhill 9.99/19.99
- New Gods for a New Age—Richmond Odom 9.99
- One Man, One Woman, One Lifetime—Rabbi Reuven Bulka 7.99
- Out of Control—Brenda Scott 9.99/19.99
- Outcome-Based Education—Peg Luksik & Pamela Hoffecker 9.99
- The Parched Soul of America—Leslie Kay Hedger w/ Dave Reagan 10.99
- Please Tell Me—Tom McKenney 9.99
- Political Correctness—David Thibodaux 9.99
- Resurrecting the Third Reich—Richard Terrell 9.99
- Revival: Its Principles and Personalities—Winkie Pratney 10.99
- Trojan Horse—Brenda Scott & Samantha Smith 9.99
- The Walking Wounded—Jeremy Reynalds 9.99

*Available in Salt Series

Available at bookstores everywhere or order direct from:
Huntington House Publishers • P.O. Box 53788 • Lafayette, LA 70505
Send check/money order. For faster service use VISA/MASTERCARD.
Call toll-free 1-800-749-4009.
Add: Freight and handling, $3.50 for the first book ordered, and $.50 for
each additional book up to 5 books.